Aqua
Yoga

by Carol Beck

DRAKE PUBLISHERS INC.

NEW YORK • LONDON

Published in 1976 by
Drake Publishers Inc.
801 Second Ave.
New York, N.Y. 10017

ISBN: 0-8473-1150-3
LC: 75-36128

Printed in the United States of America

Aqua Yoga

To Paul

Acknowledgements

Many thanks to Richard Geyer for his diligence and skill in taking the under-water photographs and to the creative Richard Ebbit for most of the photographs taken above water (except where otherwise stated); to Gretchen Teague-Schoch for her exquisite illustrations; to Kathleen and Howard Dumire, Janet Friday, Loretta Humphreys, Donna Lund, and Jacqueline Marvel for giving valuable advice; to the Bigelow Spa and Mt. Lebanon Park for the use of their pools- to my AQUAYOGA students who helped me select the best of many possible exercises.

Contents

LIST OF ILLUSTRATIONS

XII AQUAYOGA

BACKWARD ARM AND LEG STRETCH

Introduction

We would be churls indeed if, having enjoyed in our dark and contemplative beginnings the sensation of being buoyed up in a warm sea, we did not in our erect earthling state keep on good and cordial terms with water as an old friend. How welcome it is to recall old times, cast off the burden of gravity, and plunge into a pool. We glide easily, or stretch out relaxed and trustful, liberated from the magnetic pull of the earth, reveling nostalgically in a recovered simple life.

Allan P. Tory: *Wonder*

This is a book about water yoga. Those who know the delights of the water—the cool refreshment of a mid - summer's dip, the exhilaration of a winter swim indoors, the fun of splashing with favorite people—will enjoy doing the easy, gentle movements of AQUAYOGA. Those who spend their pool time sitting on the wall with feet dangling may find AQUAYOGA's invitation to stretch and trim in the water irresistible. Those who must put their tension - laden shoulders to the grindstone, nervously exhausting themselves at work and at play, will learn through AQUAYOGA to relax. How reassuring it is to be reenveloped in the simple world of water, to be supported again in what was, for nine months, the first warm and relaxing recreation of life.

Definition of AQUAYOGA

The need for an easy but effective water exercise method that relaxes as it reduces prompted me to create the unique system which I call AQUAYOGA. Swimming, though an excellent exercise, does not stretch your body in the thorough, effortless way that AQUA-YOGA does. Basically, AQUAYOGA is a new, in - the - water approach to the stretching exercises of hatha yoga. I have modified a selection of these yoga exercises, and have added others, so that most of them can be done in shallow water with no previous knowledge of either yoga or swimming necessary. They can be done in an assortment of situations—as a stretching and limbering exercise session, as a relaxing break between more vigorous endurance swimming, or, with special exercises, as an at - home bathtime routine.

Advantages of AQUAYOGA

Many factors motivate us to exercise—prevention of disease, weight reduction, an increase in energy. I would like to add one more—the sheer joy of limbering and stretching your body. AQUAYOGA exercises feel good. You will enjoy doing them. AQUAYOGA contradicts those who believe that difficult goals must be strenuously won. Exercising in the water seems much easier but is often more effective than the same movements on land. The water's buoyancy minimizes the pull of gravity for an exhilarating freedom of movement, an almost weightless but secure feeling as you move in ways more difficult or even impossible on land. The water's resistance generally requires your muscles to work 30 to 40 percent harder than they do out of the water. This muscular effort not only burns up more calories but also trims more efficiently than comparable land exercises without the usual feeling of muscular strain. Because each movement can be done as slowly and gently as desired, these unique exercises are suited for people of all ages and at every level of fitness. Unlike sports such as tennis and golf, which develop one side of the body more than the other, AQUAYOGA tones both sides equally. Exercising in the water also prevents the overheated feeling so often accompanying a workout on land. Since little space is needed for any of the exercises, they can be done discreetly in a crowded pool, often without even wetting your hair.

How to do AQUAYOGA

Most AQUAYOGA exercises are done in two steps—the stretching or lift-ing motion as you inhale and the bending forward or releasing motion as you exhale. Now you have a choice: the two steps can be done as a continuous, flowing movement; or, the position reached in some of the exercises can be held for a comfortable duration. Easy exertion is the key. If your body is not flexible, begin by repeating the easiest exercises once or twice and holding them briefly. Gradually and cautiously progress to the more difficult ones. As your muscles become limber, you can be more adventurous, holding the postures for longer periods and repeating each movement more often. It never matters if you reach a final position. What is important is that your body, in your own good time, regains its youthful suppleness. What a thrill it is to watch your muscles become long and graceful as they are stretched to their maximum flexibility. Your spine, the life-axis of your body, is strengthened and properly aligned to prevent many common back problems. The resulting good posture frees your vital organs to function properly. Rather than feeling depleted after an AQUAYOGA session, you feel refreshed and energetic.

A striking contrast to these revitalizing movements are the typically fast-paced exercises done in a calisthenics class. There, with grim determination and resulting tension, you strive to complete an entire exercise. Success is measured by whether you ever do touch your toes or master a backbend. With that accomplished, you hasten to the next exercise, still tense, still driven on to succeed, as your body is sapped of its vital energy.

Organization of the Book

Part One of this book discusses hatha yoga and the beneficial effects correct breathing, good posture and relaxation have on exercising, whether in or out of the water. Part Two includes a list of general instructions and the exercises. Essentially, an AQUAYOGA program consists of a few minutes of warm-up exercises from Chapter 6, varied stretching movements from Chapter 7 and a selection of appropriate spot reducing exercises from Chapter 8. A thorough session can be done in fifteen to twenty minutes. Swimmers will enjoy the floating and underwater exercises in Chapter 9. When no pool or lake is available, the exercises in Chapter 10 can be done at home in the bath or backyard wading pool. The practice schedules in Chapter 11 may help you to develop an AQUAYOGA program at first, but soon sheer pleasure and sensitivity to your body's needs will motivate you to move in ways most beneficial to you.

AQUAYOGA is exciting, beautifying, relaxing, and strengthening to body and mind. It will naturally proportion your figure and bring your body to the peak of physical efficiency. With a suppleness of body comes a mind enthusiastically receptive to new ideas. Emotions become more stable and balanced, less dependent on the conflicts of the external world. The well - being and relaxation that comes from doing the exercises, like a non-alcoholic, undrugged happy hour, will permeate the rest of your day. Gladness becomes an easy habit.

Treat yourself to these effective, natural AQUAYOGA movements. You will be delighted with the results.

Part One

Chapter 1
Hatha Yoga

Definition

Yoga is a systematic study of physical, mental and spiritual self - knowledge and awareness which has remained basically unchanged since its origin in India thousands of years ago. The first step usually taken in this self - discovery is hatha yoga, the science of elevating the human body to the peak of physical perfection and the mind to a state of blissful relaxation. Other systems of yoga emphasize devotional, intellectual, and meditative practice. Hatha yoga strives to reconcile the two different forces existing within us: *ha* (sun in Sanskrit, the ancient language of India), our passionate, aggressive right side; and *tha* (moon), our calm, cool left side. Yoga (to join together) unites these two opposing forces into an harmonious whole, a unity fostering both physical and mental well - being.

Hatha yoga consists of cleansing, breathing, and stretching exercises. The cleansing exercise included in this book is the Abdominal Lift in Chapter 8; the breathing techniques are explained in Chapter 3. But the stretching exercises *(asanas)* in Chapter 7 are probably the best known aspect of yoga. These superior gymnastic exercises stretch the spine in four different directions—forward, backward, in a twisting motion, and sideward. Since your complete nervous system originates in the spinal column, maintaining spinal flexibility not only keeps your body physically well but also relaxes your nerves and emotions. Those who have done hatha yoga on land know the serenity and glowing health these exercises bring. For neophytes, AQUAYOGA is a good first step since the water often makes it easier to assume positions that may seem awkward on land.

Stretching into a certain position and remaining still while holding it is the essence of yoga. Each stretch is generally repeated two or three times. There are exercises for standing, sitting, lying down, and inverting your body, as in the Head Stand and Shoulder Stand. Together they manipulate your spine and stretch your muscles to produce a healthy nervous system and a youthful limberness. Whereas many physical activities like calisthenics and competitive sports develop only the external muscles, yoga positions also massage the internal organs and glands. Most calisthenics are done mechanically without much thought; yoga stresses concentration on the muscles and parts of the spine being stretched.

Figure 1-1

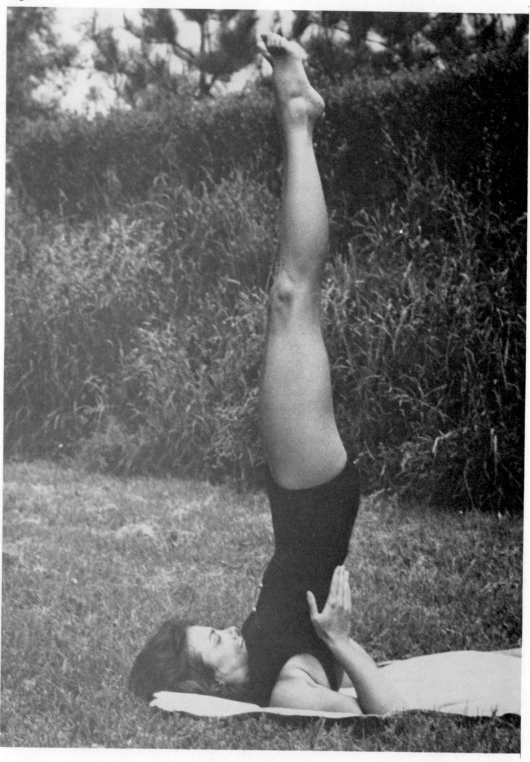

Shoulder Stand

Many of the hatha yoga positions have been modified in this book so they can be done in the water where the buoyancy and resistance of the water enhance these already effective exercises, often producing better results. But the inverted positions, the Shoulder Stand and the Head Stand, are better done out of the water.

Anyone with high blood pressure, neck problems, or heart trouble should not do the Shoulder Stand. Begin this marvelous exercise by relaxing on your back with your straight legs together and your arms at your sides, palms down. Slowly lift your legs until they are perpendicular to the floor. Press your hands downward against the floor to raise your hips. Bring your feet back behind your head. With your elbows resting on the floor, prop your hands against your back and slowly straighten your legs to a vertical position. (Figure 1-1) As your flexibility increases, you will be able to straighten your spine to the point of resting entirely on your shoulders, neck and head so that your body forms a right angle with your head. In this position, relax your legs and feet (no pointed toes), your face, your shoulders, and your spine as much as possible. Breathe rhythmically and deeply, as you enjoy being upside down. Try holding this position for one minute at first, gradually increasing the holding time to three or four minutes.

Return to the starting position by slowly bringing your knees to your forehead. Place your arms down at your sides,

Figure 1-2

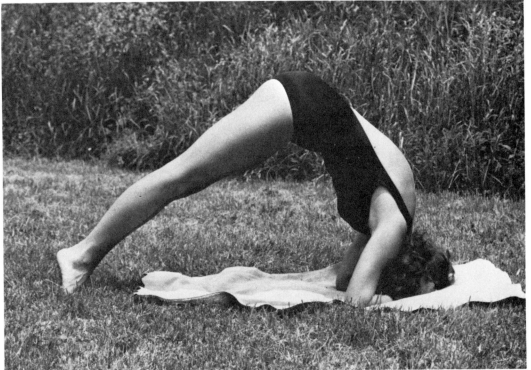

palms down, and slowly uncoil your spine to the floor, tilting your head back slightly as you come down. Place the soles of your feet on the floor and slide your legs down to rest. Relax completely on your back with your feet comfortably apart and your arms at your sides, palms up, to absorb the tranquilizing effect of this exercise. The Shoulder Stand can be done once or twice daily. This excellent position reverses the effects of gravity. It relieves the pressure on the veins of your legs while bathing the glands and organs of your upper body in extra blood. Pressing your chin against your chest while in this position stimulates your thyroid gland which energizes your entire system and regulates your appetite. In many cases, body weight is normalized, especially in those who need to lose weight. Facial circulation is increased to help prevent wrinkles and to tone your eyes, ears, hair, and even your brain. The Shoulder Stand is a tremendous rejuvenator of your entire body.

Figure 1-3

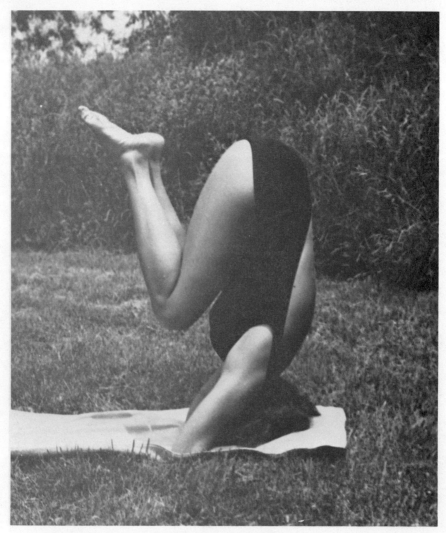

Head Stand

Although the Head Stand is the king of the yoga exercises, those with neck problems, high blood pressure or weak eye capillaries should not do it. Be sure to begin gradually, following the directions well. At first, practice in a corner as close to the wall as your hands and elbows permit. If you lose your balance, you will fall down in the same direction you came up and lessen the chance of injuring yourself.

Begin by kneeling on a soft blanket and placing your elbows on the floor in front of you with each hand holding the opposite upper arm. Now your elbows are the proper distance apart. Without moving them, slide your hands forward and interlace your fingers with your palms toward your feet. Your hands and arms are forming a firm tripod which will support the rest of your body. Place the top of your head on the floor with the back of your head resting against the palms of your hands. Push up with your toes to straighten your legs behind you so that your weight is now primarily resting on your arms, hands, and toes. (Figure 1-2) This is an exercise of its own in which you derive some of the benefits of the Head Stand. Slowly walk toward your chest until your feet are as close to your body as possible. Then gently bend your knees to your chest as you raise your feet off the floor. (Figure 1-3) Concentrate on supporting your weight primarily with your arms and hands rather than with your head. Only when you feel secure and balanced in this first step should you slowly straighten your feet up into the Head Stand. (Figure 1-4) Otherwise, begin again to walk toward your chest until your body learns that trick of balancing on head and arms.

Slowly come out of the Head Stand the same way you went up, bringing your knees to your chest and gently placing your feet on the floor. Sit back on your heels and relax with your head down for at least one minute before standing or sitting up. The wonderful therapeutic effects of the Head Stand are similar to the Shoulder Stand. The thyroid gland is not stimulated as much but every other part of your body is more intensely toned than in the Shoulder Stand.

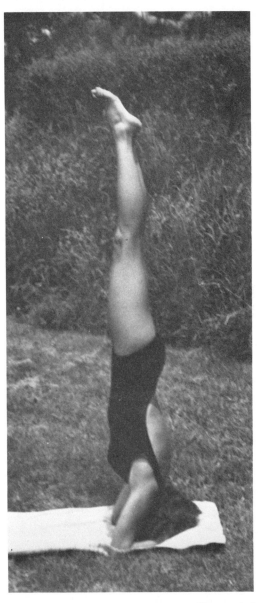

Figure 1-4

Chapter 2
Tension and Relaxation

Remedies for Tension

Everyone has periods of tension, worry, and anxiety. The general response to this stress is muscular contraction. Some people have so tightened their muscles that they unknowingly remain in a perpetual state of physical tension, tension often forceful enough to cause pain. Flexibility and relaxation are the two simple antidotes to this problem. Any kind of stretching is the most penetrating and lasting way of acquiring flexibility and eliminating muscular tension. AQUAYOGA stretches have the extra advantage of being a thorough system done in the naturally relaxing element of water. Two other natural ways of relieving tension are through the breathing exercises in Chapter 3 and the Deep Relaxation Exercise described later in this chapter.

Tension as a Lifestyle

To understand the impact tension has, consider the lifestyle of the most nervous person you know. His body has probably become rigid from lack of exercise; his tight muscles keep him in a constant state of physical tension. He habitually clenches his jaws, hunches his shoulders and wrinkles his forehead. On those rare occasions when he sits still, he wraps his legs nervously around his chair. When he drives, he grips the steering wheel too tightly. His life is so structured that he lacks the looseness to do anything spontaneously. In fact, his whole being is rigid to life's inevitable changes and adjustments. He has lost the natural ability to relax. In an effort to escape an anxiety-ridden existence, he races through each day, scurrying from one activity to the next, dulling his mind into a numb forgetfulness, a retreat from his careworn self. Even his leisure time is spent hastening from the golf course to the garden. His restless living only leads to more restlessness. His body eventually protests with a most effective weapon—illness. Unfortunately, he is not alone in his inability to relax. Look around you at those plagued by worries and fears. Recall the people whose aching backs, insomnia, and chronic depressions are all a result of tension to realize the need for relaxation—not the attention - diverting activities often thought of as relaxation, such as smoking, drinking, or watching television—but a consciously learned system of actively relaxing every part of your body.

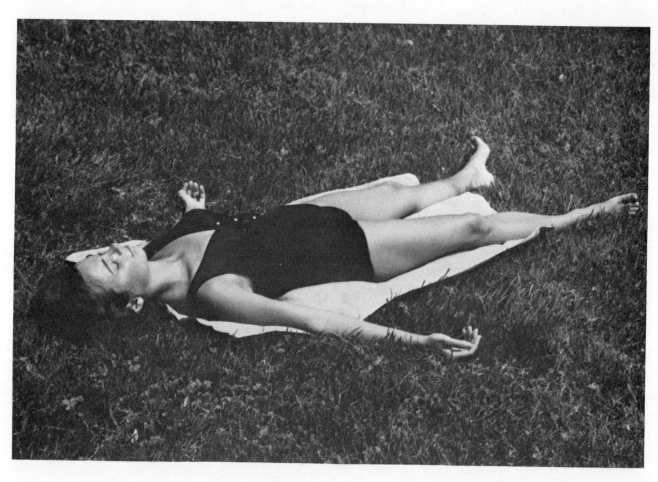

Figure 2-1

Deep Relaxation Exercise

Think of tension as a stubborn and potentially dangerous rash. If you promptly apply the proper treatment, the rash will disappear rather than develop into something more serious. The same is true of tension. If it is alleviated when it occurs, it will not mushroom into an ineradicable disease that consumes your body as well as your mind. The Deep Relaxation Exercise is a valuable aid to relieving tension. This technique of consciously relaxing every part of your body may take five or ten minutes at first. Once you know how completely relaxed muscles feel, you can use this method to relax at will at any time in any position. To replenish your body with energy so you will feel refreshed after your exercise period, be sure to follow each AQUAYOGA session with this delightful technique. Whatever time you choose to do it, you may soon reach a level of relaxation you never knew existed.

Deep Relaxation can be practiced in any comfortable position. When first learning it, begin by lying on your back with your feet comfortably apart and your arms slightly away from your sides, palms facing up. (Figure 2-1) This is the Corpse (sometimes less bleakly called the Sponge). To acquire conscious control of your muscles—deliberate tensing develops the control that makes deliberate relaxing possible—alternately tense and then relax parts of your body beginning with your legs and progressing upward to your face. Begin with your right leg raised a few inches. Tense it firmly while keeping the rest of your body relatively relaxed. Then release the tension as you drop your leg limply to the floor. Alternately raise, tense, and relax your other leg, your arms, your buttocks, and your chest (arch your back slightly). Tense your face by grimacing and squeez-

ing your eyes tightly together; then relax your face into a smooth serenity. Gently roll your head from side to side before resting it comfortably in the center. Consciously relax each part of your body from your feet to your head by thinking "My feet are relaxing, my ankles are relaxing," until you reach "My scalp is relaxing, my brain is relaxing." Lie quietly as you linger for at least several minutes in this peaceful state. Calm your mind by watching your breath, which becomes slower, deeper and more rhythmical as you concentrate on it. For a gentle transition from this delightful state of relaxation back to a more active state, slowly stretch before rising as a cat does when it first awakens. Your stamina and energy level afterward will be noticeably increased since deep relaxation relieves fatigue in minutes often more effectively than several hours of sleep. Do not be discouraged if complete relaxation is difficult at first. Any relaxation is better than none. Gradually you will learn this marvelous technique until what is at first a time-consuming practice becomes possible immediately.

Self - Awareness

Once you have experienced what true relaxation is, your sensitivity to unnecessary tension in your body is heightened. Check yourself now to see how relaxed your legs and face are. Or have you so habitually tensed those muscles that they remain tight even when you are not using them? Like an efficiency expert in the use of energy, you will gradually eliminate this wasted effort and selectively tense only those muscles needed while the rest of your body remains relaxed. You will not complicate a naturally easy movement by grasping your pen too tightly when writing or tensing your face as you do leg exercises.

The feeling of serenity and peacefulness experienced after deep relaxation can easily be extended into the rest of the day. Make a list of everything in your day that makes you tense. Eliminate what you reasonably can; put some ease into a too hectic schedule. By slowing down that killing pace and having gentler self-expectations, you allow yourself the pleasure of the present moment. So much of our culture stresses accomplishments in the future—saving for a rainy day, working hard for a promotion—that we often forget to be fully aware of what we are doing this minute, now. Acting with complete awareness of everything you do—whether it is stretching and bending, opening a door, eating, or loving—enables you to experience the fullness of life in the present. And it is in the present, not in the future, where life is to be had.

Your relaxed mind will not only be more aware but will also dwell less on negative thoughts. Instead of coloring your world with stories of misfortune and bad luck, the blissful feeling of relaxation helps you to emphasize the positive aspects of life. With the serene mind acquired by learning to relax your body, you are more inclined to positively accept the world around you. You begin to realize that happiness is not dependent on external events but only on your reaction to them. Happiness is, after all, a state of mind.

Chapter 3
Breathing Techniques

Incorrect Breathing

Breathing is often a function occurring only in your chest with your diaphragm and rib cage remaining still. The shallow intake of oxygen and outgo of carbon dioxide that this chest breathing provides often uses only 1/3 of your lung capacity, fulfilling only 1/10 of your oxygen needs. Residual air with carbon dioxide lies in your lungs like stagnant water. Your cells, especially those of the central nervous system, are starved of the oxygen they require for proper functioning. This oxygen insufficiency is often the cause of chronic fatigue and depression. Your diaphragm and rib cage grow rigid from disuse. An interesting theory proposes that this rigidity reflects certain psychological states: inadequate inhalation represents the fear of living positively and assertively; insufficient exhalation signifies the inability to relax and openly express true feelings.

Deep Breathing

Deep breathing, in which your abdomen, rib cage, and chest expand and contract, fills your lungs completely from bottom to top rather than just the top as in chest breathing. It can have surprising physical, emotional, and mental benefits. Your complexion glows; your eyes sparkle. Your diaphragm and rib cage become flexible. The millions of bone, nerve, blood, and tissue cells, which are so dependent upon a good supply of oxygen for proper functioning, are well nourished. Oxygen stimulates your entire circulatory system, purifying it and keeping it ready for emergencies and strain. Because deep breathing revitalizes every organ and system of your body, it tends to increase resistance to disease. The ancient yogis conjectured that deep breathing not only aided relaxation but prolonged life as well. Using animals as examples, they observed that shallow breathers like mice and rabbits were nervous animals with short life spans, whereas those who breathed deeply, like parrots and elephants, lived longer.

Deep breathing is also the natural way to control emotions. Have you ever noticed how closely related your emotional states are to your rate of breathing? Your breath tends to be fast, uneven, and high in your chest when excited. Short inhalations and long exhalations, as in sighing, characterize depression. During intense concentration, breathing often momentarily stops. Not only does your breathing reflect your emotional state, but it can influence it as well. Holding your breath is a sure way of causing ten- sion, whereas slow, rhythmic breathing produces a calm, serene mood. With slow, deep breathing you can also alleviate tension, anger, and depression. Like a natural high, deep breathing helps you to feel good again.

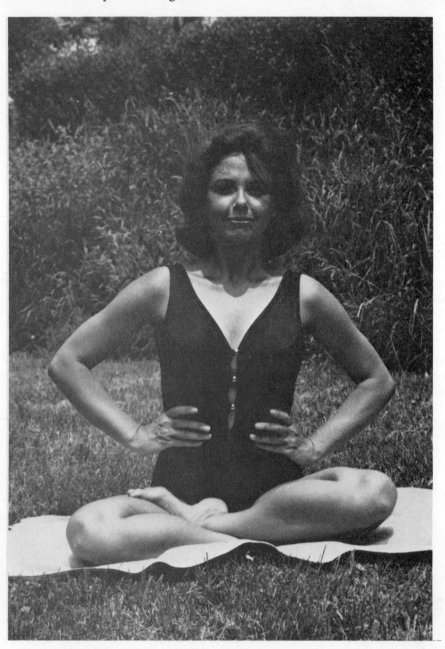

Figure 3-1

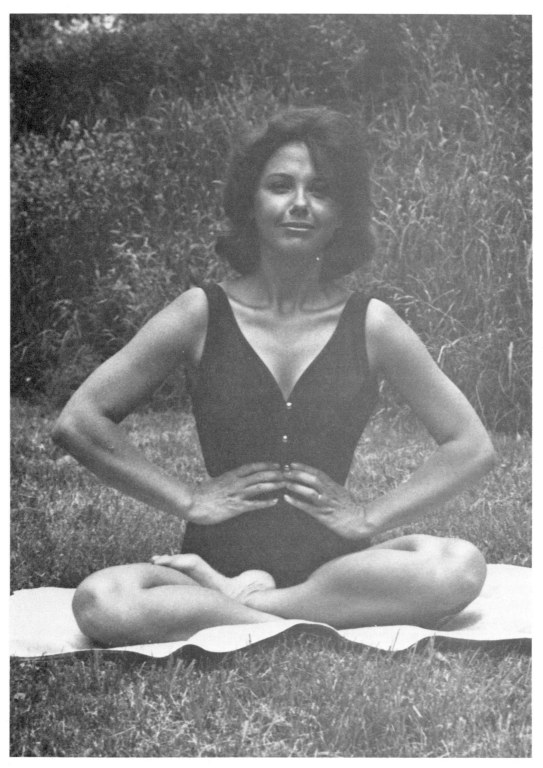

Figure 3-2

Deep Breathing Exercise

The remedy for habitual shallow breathing is almost too simple to be believed. In any comfortable sitting, standing, or reclining position (the latter is a good learning position), place your hands lightly against your lower ribs with your middle fingers touching in the center and your elbows pointed out to the sides. The rib area is where you should feel the most movement as you breathe deeply. Inhale through your nose and expand your ribs sideways like an accordion so that your hands move farther apart. Your abdomen and chest will also gently expand. There is no need to lift your shoulders. (Figure 3-1) Exhale, also through your nose, as your ribs narrow again. (Figure 3-2) Your abdomen, which naturally tends to contract with each exhalation, should be pulled in as well. This expansion and contraction of your abdomen is the most efficient method of filling your lungs with oxygen. Allowing your abdomen to expand while inhaling lowers your diaphragm to fill the bottom of your lungs with air. Contracting your abdomen while exhaling raises your diaphragm, enabling it to act like a squeezing pump to help expel air from your lungs. Watch a sleeping baby for a perfect demonstration of this natural breathing method.

Repeat this Deep Breathing Exercise two or three consecutive times at first, completely ventilating your lungs as you inhale and contracting your ribs and your abdominal muscles as you exhale. Loosen tight belts, bras or other restrictive clothing to permit free expansion of your ribs. Your body may be unaccustomed to so much oxygen, so be cautious. If you do hyperventilate, take a few steps or swing your arms back and forth to expend oxygen. Later in the day repeat the deep breathing exercise several times until your body becomes accustomed to the extra oxygen. You can slowly increase your practice time to ten or twenty minutes if you desire. Remember that this is only an exercise. Although it will gradually change your normal, subconscious breathing into a deeper, slower and healthier pattern, do not try to breathe this way all the time.

Alternate Nostril Breathing

Alternate Nostril Breathing is another simple and natural exercise utilizing the vital fuel of oxygen to calm your central nervous system and provide you with more energy. It is an especially soothing technique often used by performers to relieve stage fright. Begin by sitting, standing, or lying down in any comfortable position with your spine in good alignment. Close your right nostril with your right thumb and inhale only through your left nostril as you count to eight. Close your left nostril with your ring finger—your forefinger and middle finger are resting lightly on your forehead—and hold both nostrils closed for a count of four. Then slowly exhale through your right nostril for a count of eight. Continue by inhaling through your right nostril, holding your breath and exhaling through your left nostril. When you have done all that, you have completed one round of breathing. At first you may be comfortable doing only three or four rounds. Those who have gradually accustomed themselves to the increase in oxygen often enjoy doing Alternate Nostril Breathing for 15 to 30 minutes at a time. But even four rounds daily strengthen and calm your nervous system, producing an habitual serenity in almost any situation. Doing it in snatches throughout the day—outside in the warm sun and fresh air is especially delightful—will help you to replace negative emotions like fear and worry with an even-temperedness and peacefulness. Six or seven rounds while lying in bed at night is a great aid to curing insomnia and guaranteeing a relaxed sleep that leaves you energetic and refreshed the next morning.

Coordinated Breathing

Coordinating your breath with the AQUAYOGA exercises results in better control over everything you do in the water. Inhaling brings an element lighter than water to your body to support activity as you rise toward the surface. Exhaling decreases buoyancy, helping you to sink. Generally you inhale during the more strenuous action or as you stretch or raise any part of your body, and exhale with any movement requiring abdominal contraction or as you release or relax. For instance, you would inhale to raise your legs in the water and exhale to lower them. This synchronized breathing, stressed throughout the book, produces a certain basic rhythm which relaxes your nervous system and makes the movement itself more graceful and beautiful. Although the inhalation and exhalation are usually done through your nostrils with your mouth closed, you may want to part your lips slightly to prevent water from getting into your nose. Coordinated breathing may require conscious effort at first, but it soon becomes automatic.

Chapter 4
Good Posture

Its Importance

Good posture makes you feel as vibrantly alive and self - assured as you look. On the other hand, chronically slumped shoulders, protruding abdomen, thickening waistline, and drooping head show the world that you are either lazy, unhealthy, or lacking self - confidence. These signs of poor posture also put added stress on your spine and generally indicate that you have lost the battle with that ever - insistent but invisible force—gravity.

Three Important Steps

Specifically, there are three easy steps to naturally aligning and balancing your body, for an instantly slimmer, more beautiful appearance. To reinforce good postural habits, do these three simple steps often during your AQUAYOGA sessions as well as throughout the day. Begin by standing with your feet pointed straight ahead, a shoulder width apart, your knees slightly bent and your arms relaxed at your side. Tuck your buttocks together and under as if to avoid a spank-

ing as you pull your abdomen in and up. (The Abdominal Lift in Chapter 8 is excellent for acquiring this kind of control.) With your pelvic girdle tucked in tightly, stretch your ribs and the crown of your head up away from your hips as if reaching for the ceiling or sky. With your shoulders relaxed and down, inch them backward. Your arms are still relaxed at your sides. Think often of these three reminders—"tuck, lift, and relaxed shoulders back." Remember that proper body alignment is not a static, affected carriage but rather a dynamic, natural way of holding your body whatever you are doing, whether sitting at the dinner table, walking to the office, or playing tennis. What at first may seem awkward will gradually become natural as you learn to tune into this new way of holding yourself.

Shoulder - level water is the easiest place to begin this "tuck, lift, and relaxed shoulders back" stance since at this depth your body feels so much lighter than on land. Here you can also detect any faulty patterns in gait as you walk in slow, underwater motion. An effective way to bring about postural changes is to gradually walk into shallower water; maintaining correct posture becomes progressively harder as you give up the support of the water for the force of gravity.

Figure 4-1

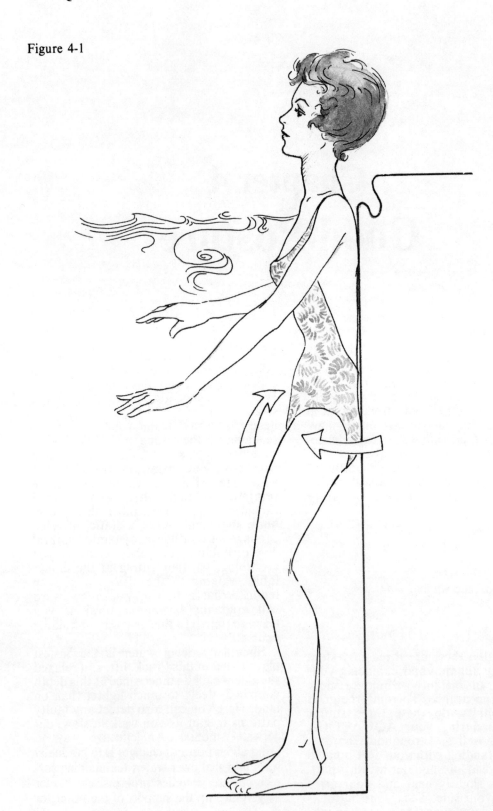

Pelvic Tuck Exercise

Benefits of Good Posture

The following exercise, which helps you to acquire and strengthen the pelvic tuck, should also be done in shoulder - level water. Stand with your back against the pool wall, your feet six to ten inches away from the wall and six inches apart. With your knees bent slightly, tuck in your buttocks and, exhaling, tighten your abdomen in order to press your back at your waistline against the wall. (Figure 4-1) Hold for a count of six and then inhale, relaxing your abdomen and buttocks as your lower back hollows away from the wall. Besides being the key to proper body alignment, this exercise trims your abdomen and strengthens your lower back. It can be repeated ten to twenty times.

The rewards of good posture are many. The pelvic tuck, in which your buttocks are pulled under and your abdomen is tightened, is a strong muscular girdle which positions your vital organs naturally. Habitually holding in this pelvic girdle also prevents intervertebral disc problems. Lifting your rib cage inhibits an accumulation of fat on your hips, allows for the healthful functioning of your heart and lungs and strengthens the muscles of your middle back. Stretching the top of your head up with your neck long and straight relieves tension in the back of your neck and often causes multiple chins to disappear.

Part Two

Chapter 5
General Instructions for Doing AQUAYOGA

Follow these simple directions for a successful and enjoyable AQUAYOGA session.

1. Wait the traditional hour after a meal before exercising.

2. Become accustomed to the water by entering the pool slowly and splashing water on your arms and shoulders before totally immersing.

3. The exercises are divided into three groups—(a) warmups (b) stretches, and (c) spot reducers.

   (a) Warm up with assorted jumping, running and kicking exercises from Chapter 6.

   (b) Do the forward, backward, sideward, and twisting stretching movements from Chapter 7 slowly with a calm attitude. Many of the positions stretched into can be held in stillness for a comfortable duration as you breathe deeply. Concentrate on and enjoy the stretching taking place. These exercises are meant to relax you so never force yourself into any position. Remember it is the practicing, not the position reached, which is important. Always stop when you are tired or uncomfortable.

   (c) The spot reducing exercises from Chapter 8 are best done at a quick pace. The faster you move in the water, the harder your muscles must work against the water's resistance. This extra muscular effort trims more efficiently than slower movements or often the same movement on land.

4. Unless otherwise stated, do each exercise in chest - to shoulder - level water.

5. As a general rule, repeat each exercise three to six times although you may work up to ten or twenty times with your favorite spot reducing exercises.

6. You can create your own schedule of

AQUAYOGA exercises, choosing one or two movements from each of the four ways to stretch your spine and adding the warm-ups and spot reducing exercises that suit your needs, or you can choose the schedule most appropriate for you from Chapter 11.

7. During your AQUAYOGA session, take relaxation breaks every four or five minutes by resting your back against the pool wall with your feet comfortably away and your arms floating forward and up.

8. Always maintain proper spinal alignment as explained in Chapter 4, by tucking your buttocks together and in, tightening your abdomen, and lifting your torso and the crown of your head up.

9. Coordinating your breathing with the exercises as explained in Chapter 3 not only makes movement easier but also has a soothing effect on your central nervous system. Both the inhalation and exhalation are done through your nose, but you may want to keep your mouth open slightly to prevent water from entering your nostrils. If you find coordinated breathing awkward, do just the exercises alone first. When they are familiar enough to you, breathe with them by inhaling during the more strenuous part of the movement or as you stretch or lift up, and exhaling as you return to the starting position or as you bend down. Gradually, this breathing becomes automatic, requiring no conscious effort at all.

10. The directive to "hold at poolside" will differ according to the pool you are using. If your pool does not have a ledge or bracket six to ten inches below the top of the wall for you to grasp, you may find it easier to hold the bars of the ladder for support.

11. If you are unaccustomed to exercising, begin gradually.

12. Nonswimmers should always stay near the side of the pool when exercising.

13. If you have any medical problems or if any exercise causes you intense pain, consult your doctor before continuing. You will gradually learn to distinguish between the healthy, beneficial feeling of stretching out tight muscles and the real pain that is your body's warning signal that something serious is wrong.

14. Warm water in the low eighties is an ideal temperature for relaxing your muscles and making them more stretchable. If your pool water is cool, intersperse a few brisk warm-ups and spot reducing exercises among the slower stretching ones to avoid being chilled.

15. Since many of the AQUAYOGA exercises can be done out of the water with little or no modification, you can maintain a regular exercise program even when not in a pool. Do the exercises regularly either in the pool where the water's buoyancy and resistance will make them often more

effective or on land when no pool is available.

16. After your AQUAYOGA session, relax out of the pool on your back for five or ten minutes with the Deep Relaxation Exercise in Chapter 2.

Chapter 6
Warm-up Exercises

These light, conditioning exercises literally warm up your body's deep muscle temperature. By increasing your circulation, they also help you adjust more quickly to cool water.

All of the warm - up exercises should be done in a continuous, flowing motion. Each one can be repeated for one to two minutes or until you are comfortably exerted. Five minutes of any assortment of walking, kicking, and jumping exercises is sufficient preparation for the more intensive stretching to follow.

Walking Exercises

Raised Leg Walk

—trims your thighs, abdomen and buttocks

Stand away from poolside, with your feet together and your arms forward at shoulder level, palms down.

Figure 6-1

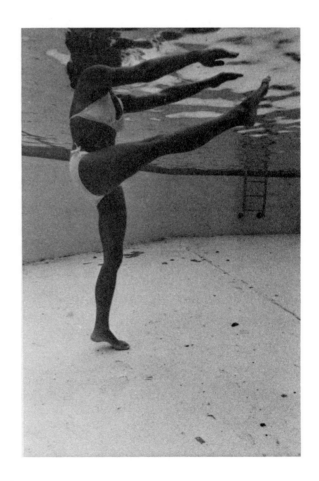

Inhale, raising your right knee to your arms and then straightening your leg to touch your foot to your hands. (Figure 6-1) Flex your heel for a more effective leg stretch.

Exhale, lowering your straight leg to the pool floor.

Walk, raising alternate legs for one to two minutes.

On Land: Same

Knee Lift

—increases flexibility in your hip and thigh muscles
Standing in good posture with your feet together, hug alternate bent knees to your chest for one to two minutes. (Figure 6-2)

On Land: Same

Jogging

—increases your endurance
—trims your abdomen

Run on the balls of your feet, raising alternate knees high toward your chest as if you were prancing. Keep your back straight and your abdomen and buttocks tucked in.

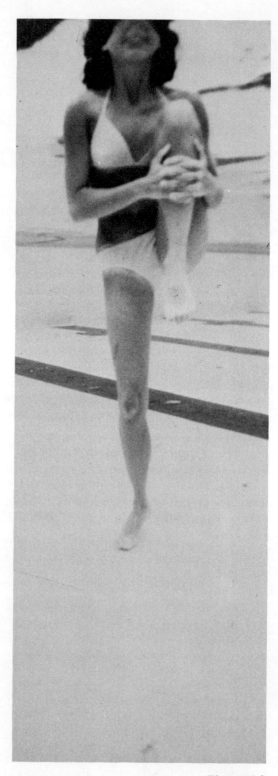

Figure 6-2

Continue until pleasantly invigorated.

Vary the movement by jogging backwards.

On Land: Same

Soldier Walk

   —tones your arms
   —trims your thighs, calves and hips
Stand away from poolside with your feet together and your arms at your sides. Your legs remain straight throughout.

Inhale, raising your right leg and your left arm forward so they are parallel to the pool floor. Your raised heel and wrist are flexed (Figure 6-3).

Exhale, in a continuous motion, lowering your right leg and left arm as you raise your alternate arm and leg forward.

Continue this stiff-legged walk for one to two minutes.

On Land: Same

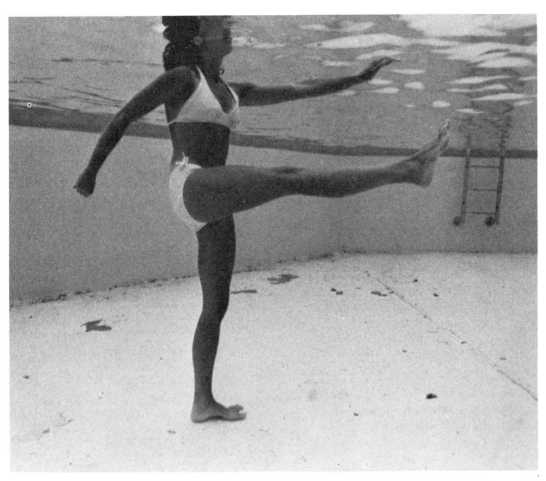

Figure 6-3

Foot Variation

—strengthens and limbers your feet and ankles

Keeping your abdomen and buttocks tucked in tightly, the crown of your head high, and your shoulders back and relaxed, walk with your feet in the following positions:

on your toes and then on your heels;

on the inside of your feet and then on the outside of your feet;

with your toes pointed in and with your toes pointed out.

Step twenty times with each position.

On Land: Same

Skipping

—increases your endurance
Skip exhuberantly, lifting your raised knee high to your chest for several minutes.

On Land: Same

Tiptoe Walking

—trims your waistline and hips

Stand on tiptoe with your feet together and your arms overhead, palms facing each other.

Tiptoe forward on your left foot while reaching up with your left hand as if to touch the sky. Step forward on your right foot and reach with your right hand. Move your ribcage up by holding your body straight without tilting to the side for an excellent stretch to your hips and waistline.

Continue for several minutes.

On Land: Same

Kicking Exercises

Flutter Kick

—trims your legs and hips
Facing the wall and holding at poolside, let your straight legs float up behind you. With your knees relaxed but not bent, your ankles flexible and toes pointed, kick briskly in small arcs of eighteen to twenty - four inches.
Repeat for one to two minutes.
Vary the kick by lying on your back with your hands holding at poolside.

On Land: Not practical

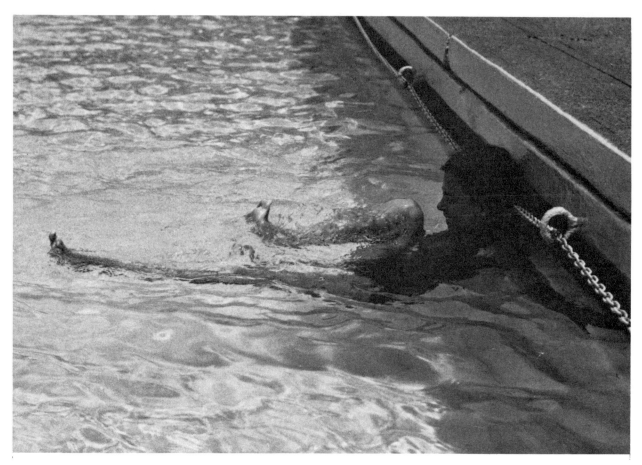

Figure 6-4

Leg Push - Out   Bicycle Kick

—firms your abdomen
—increases circulation in your legs
With your back to the wall and your arms and hands holding at poolside, bend your knees to your chest. With heels leading, thrust alternate feet forward as if to push a float away as you draw your opposite knee to your chest. Keep your abdominal muscles tight. (Figure 6-4)
Continue for one to two minutes.
On Land: Not Practical

—reduces your abdomen and hips
With your back to the wall and your hands holding at poolside, let your legs float forward and up. Pedal a bicycle in the water, bringing alternate feet out of the water with each kick and then vigorously kicking downward. Try reversing the motion for a good lesson in coordination.
Continue for one to two minutes.
This kick can also be done lying on your

side with one hand holding at poolside and the other against the wall, fingers pointing down, for support.

On Land: Begin by either lying on your back with your hands, palms down, under your buttocks, or by raising your back off the floor into the Shoulder Stand (Chapter 1). Pedal a bicycle with your legs.

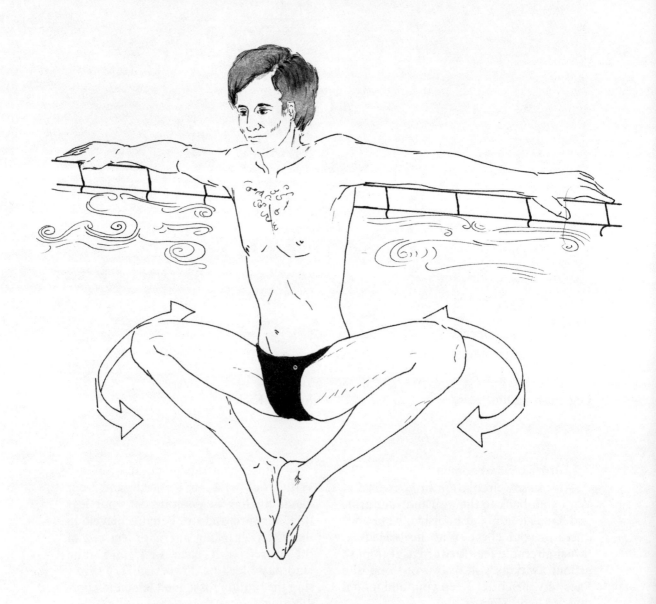

Figure 6-5

Butterfly

—trims your inner thighs

With your back to the wall and your arms and hands holding at poolside, bend your knees to your chest and then part them with the soles of your feet together. Concentrate on using your inner thigh muscles as you flutter your knees back and forth like butterfly wings for one to two minutes. The soles of your feet stay together throughout. (Figure 6-5)

On Land: Sitting with your knees bent and the soles of your feet together close to your body, flutter your knees up and down.

Jump Kick

—trims your abdomen
—increases your endurance

Stand with your back to the wall, feet together, and your hands holding at poolside. Jump and kick, chorus style, raising alternate straight legs high in front of you for one to two minutes.

On Land: Same

Backward Kick

—trims your buttocks and thighs
—increases your endurance

Stand facing the wall with your feet together and your hands, a shoulder width apart, holding at poolside.

Jump and kick alternate straight legs backward for one to two minutes. (Figure 6-6).

Vary the movement by bending your knees.

On Land: Same

Figure 6-6

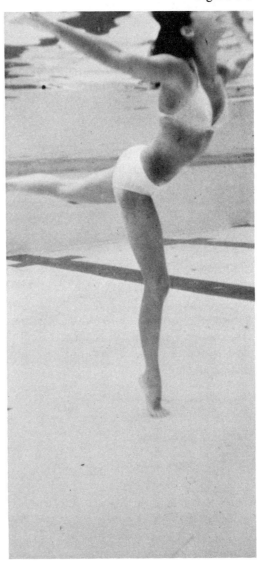

Scissors Kick

—trims your abdomen, hips and buttocks
With your back to the wall and your hands holding at poolside, let your legs float forward and up. Roll onto your left hip and kick in long back and forth motions for one to two minutes. Reverse by rolling onto your right hip and kicking.
Vary the movement by lying on your side with one hand holding at poolside and the other braced lower against the pool wall, fingers pointing down. Kick your legs back and forth in a scissors movement parallel to the water's surface.
Swimmers' Variation: Suspended in deep water, with your right side to the wall, hold with your right hand at poolside. Let your left arm float to the side at shoulder level. With your toes pointed toward the pool floor, kick in rapid back and forth movements.
On Land: Lie on your right side with your right arm stretched overhead and your left hand on the floor in front of you. Your legs are straight and together. Raise your legs several inches from the floor and scissors kick in rapid back and forth movements.

Jumping Exercises

Hopping

—increases your circulation
—tones your entire body
Stand away from poolside with your feet

close together, your knees slightly bent and your arms at your sides.
Hop quickly across the pool. Keep your buttocks and abdomen tucked in tightly, your shoulders back and relaxed and the crown of your head high. Spring higher as your strength increases.
Continue for one to two minutes.
Swimmers' Variation: Exhale, clapping your hands together overhead as you submerge into a squatting position with your feet together on the pool floor. Inhale, slapping your arms to your sides as you spring high out of the water. Continue bobbing for one to two minutes.
On Land: Not practical

Figure 6-7

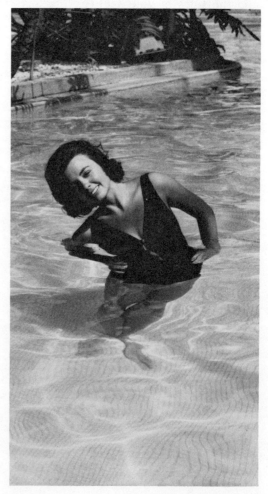

Side Jump

Leaping

—reduces your waistline
Stand away from poolside with your feet together and your hands on your hips.
Jump with both feet to the left as you stretch your torso sideways to the right. (Figure 6-7)
Reverse and repeat in a continuous motion for one to two minutes.
For a more intense sideward stretch, keep your arms overhead with palms together as you bend from side to side.
On Land: Not practical

—increases your endurance
—trims your waistline
Stand away from poolside with your feet together and your arms out to the sides at shoulder level. Keep your chest high and your arms at shoulder level throughout. Leap forward on your right foot as you twist your torso and head to the left. (Figure 6-8) Leap onto your left foot as you twist to the left.

Figure 6-8

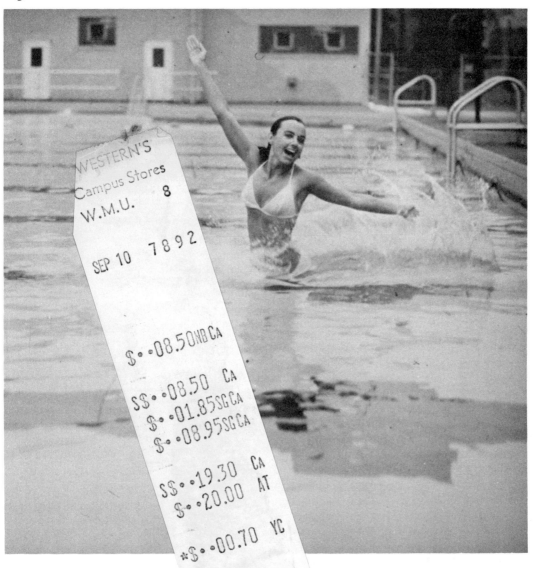

Figure 6-9

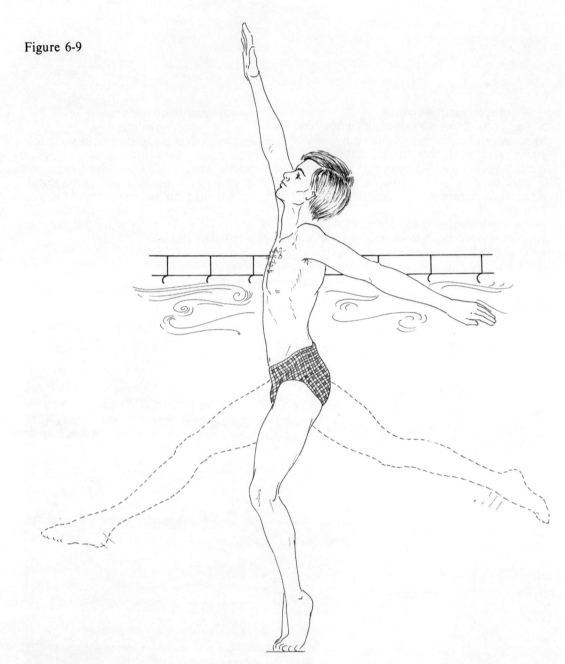

Split Jump

—trims your thighs
Stand away from poolside with your feet together and your arms at your sides.
Spring high with your right leg forward and your left leg back as you stretch your right arm overhead and your left arm back. (Figure 6-9) Land with both feet together.
Spring high again with your leg and arm positions reversed.
Continue for one to two minutes.
On Land: Not practical

Figure 6-10

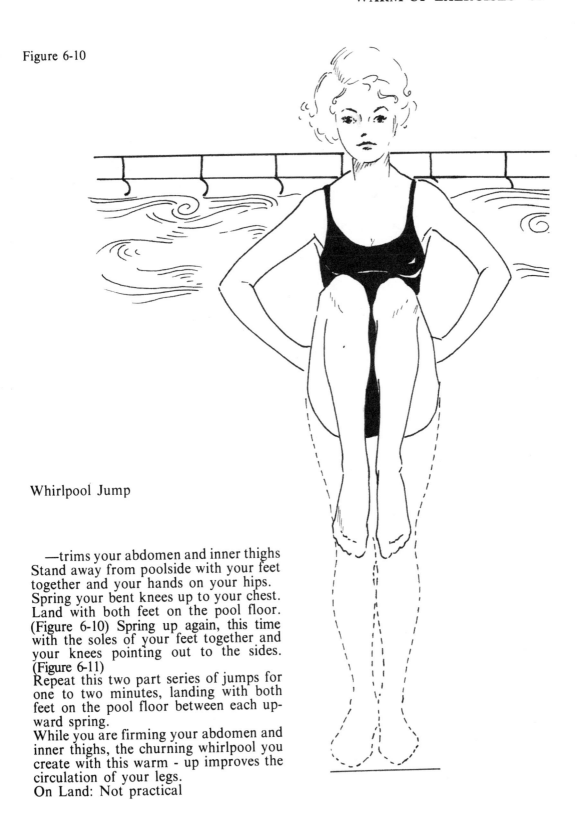

Whirlpool Jump

—trims your abdomen and inner thighs
Stand away from poolside with your feet
together and your hands on your hips.
Spring your bent knees up to your chest.
Land with both feet on the pool floor.
(Figure 6-10) Spring up again, this time
with the soles of your feet together and
your knees pointing out to the sides.
(Figure 6-11)
Repeat this two part series of jumps for
one to two minutes, landing with both
feet on the pool floor between each upward spring.
While you are firming your abdomen and
inner thighs, the churning whirlpool you
create with this warm - up improves the
circulation of your legs.
On Land: Not practical

Figure 6-11

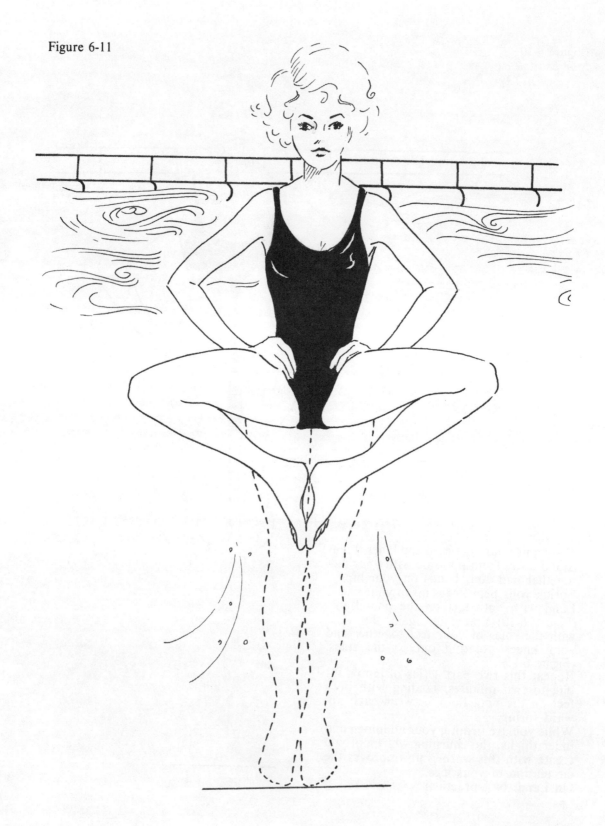

Forward Lunge

—trims your thighs and abdomen
Stand away from poolside with your feet
together and your hands on your hips.
Like a fencer, lunge with your right foot
forward and your left leg back. Both
knees are bent. Jump in place by reversing the position of your legs.

Continue with alternate feet forward for
one to two minutes.
Swimmers' Variation (Bobbing): Exhale,
clapping your hands overhead as you submerge into the forward lunge. (Figure 6-12)
Slap your arms to your sides as you
spring high out of the water and inhale. Exhale, submerging with your other foot lung-
ed forward and your arms overhead again.
Continue this excellent conditioning activity
for one to two minutes.
On Land: Not practical

Figure 6-12

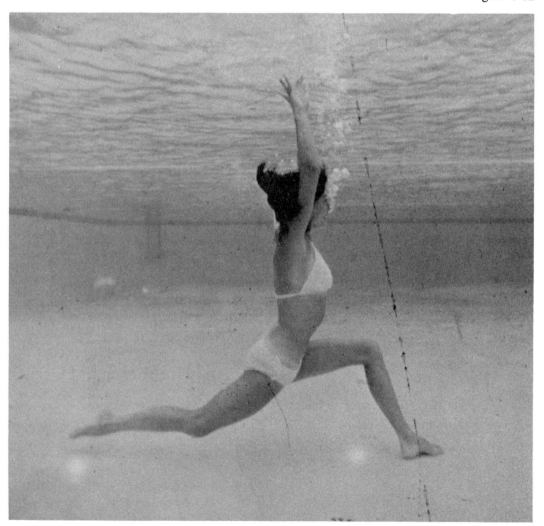

Sideward Lunge

   —increases your endurance
   —trims your thighs and hips
Stand away from poolside with your feet together and your hands on your hips. Jump and then lunge to the right like a fencer by stepping sideways with your right foot and bending your right knee. Spring high and land again with your leg position reversed.

Continue lunging from side to side for one to two minutes.
Swimmers' Variation: Exhale, clapping your arms overhead as you submerge into a sideward lunge position. Slap your arms to your sides as you spring out of the water, inhaling, and landing with both feet together. Exhale, submerging as you lunge to the other side with your arms overhead again. Continue bobbing in this manner for one to two minutes.
On Land: Not practical

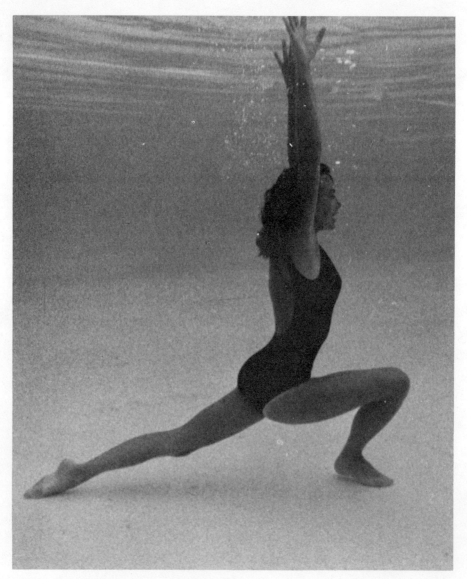

Figure 6-13

Chapter 7
Stretching Exercises

Stretching is a marvelous therapeutic activity. As you stretch your tight muscles back to their youthful elasticity, your body relaxes. As your body relaxes, your taut muscles yield more readily to tension-relieving movements. Each stretch should be done slowly with a serene attitude and need only be repeated two or three times. After you have eased into any of the following stretches, you may hold that position motionless, breathing deeply and evenly, for as long as you are comfortable. This intensifies the stretch for a more relaxing effect and often massages and stimulates your internal organs and glands.

Forward Stretching Exercises

These forward stretching exercises elongate the muscles on either side of your spine to prevent the gradual shortening which comes with age. Many of these exercises also trim your abdomen and maintain flexibility in your calf and thigh muscles. The Knee Raises, the Alternate Leg Raises and the Leg Stretch in Chapter 8 are good warm-ups for the more intensive stretches of the Wall Walk and the Head to Knee Exercise of this chapter.

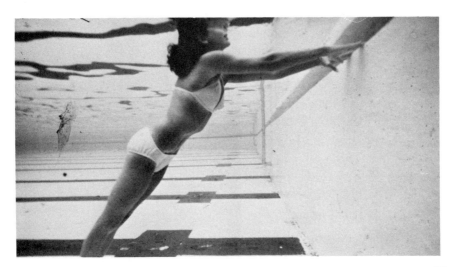

Figure 7-1

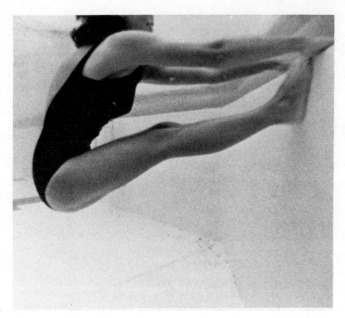

Figure 7-2

Wall Walk

—trims your abdomen
—stretches your back and leg muscles
Face the wall with your hands, a shoulder width apart, holding at poolside. Stretch your legs behind you with your feet together and flat on the pool floor, heels down.
Keeping your legs straight and heels down whenever possible, walk forward and up the wall in eight to ten short steps. The more limber your back and legs are, the higher you will go. Return by walking down and back on the pool floor again. Repeat three times.
On Land: Not practical

Wall Stretch

Figure 7-3

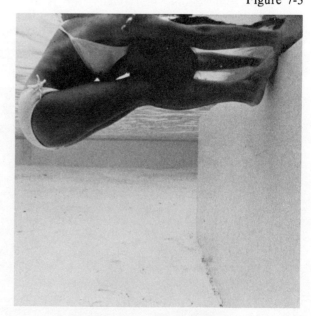

—provides a therapeutic stretch of your entire spine
Stand facing the wall an arm's length away with your feet together and your hands a shoulder width apart, holding at poolside.

Inhale, stretching your straight legs back with your pointed toes touching the floor. Keep your buttocks and abdomen tucked in. (Figure 7-1)

Exhale, placing your feet on the pool wall with your knees bent to your chest and your chin tucked between them.

Return to a standing position and repeat three times.
On Land: Not practical

Head to Knee

—trims your abdomen
—stretches and relaxes your leg and back muscles

Face the wall with both hands, a shoulder width apart, holding at poolside. Place your feet close together high on the wall with your knees bent. If your pool has no ledge or gutter to grasp, hold the bars of the ladder with your feet on the highest step comfortable for you.

Inhale, straightening your knees so that your heels are on the wall. (Figure 7-2) The higher your feet, the better the stretch. You can bounce in this position for an effective limbering of your legs and lower back. Swimmers can exhale, submerging head to knees. (Figure 7-3)

Exhale, bending your knees to your chest again.

Repeat three times.

On Land: Sit with your legs straight in front of you. Inhale, raising your arms overhead. Exhale, stretching forward to clasp whatever part of your legs you can.

Ankle to Forehead Stretch

—stretches your leg muscles
—maintains flexibility in your hip joints

Stand away from poolside with your feet together and your arms to the sides at shoulder level. Lift your right knee forward in order for your right hand to cross over your bent knee and clasp the outside of your right heel. Your right arm is underneath your right calf. Hold the outside of your right arch with your left hand.

Inhale, raising your right foot high to touch your forehead. Lean forward slightly. (Figure 7-4)

Exhale, lowering your foot.

Repeat three times with each leg.
If balance is a problem, stand with your back against the wall for support.

On Land: Sit with your legs extended straight in front of you. Clasping your right foot as in the water, press it to your forehead with both hands.

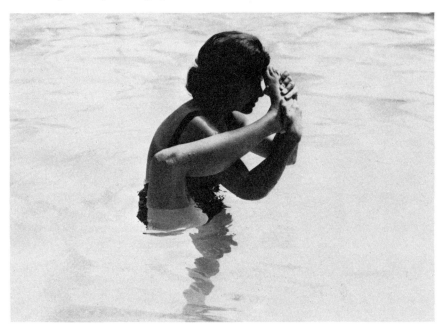

Figure 7-4

Figure 7-5

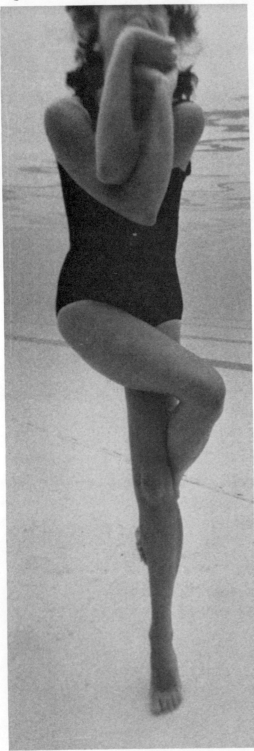

Eagle

—trims your thighs
—develops your balance
Stand away from poolside with your left
knee bent slightly so that your right leg
can wind in front of and then behind your
left calf. With elbows bent, cross your left
elbow over your right arm and clasp
hands with your left palm facing up and
your right palm facing down. Rest your
chin on your hands.

Inhale, straightening your left knee
slightly. (Figure 7-5)

Exhale, bending your left knee as if to sit.

Repeat this up and down movement three
times on each side.
This balancing position, like the Tree and
the Arm and Leg Lift, can be done in
progressively shallower water. This increases your stability to balance on land
without the support of the water.
On Land: Same. Fix your gaze on
something at eye level to help maintain
balance.

Backward Stretching Exercises

Many of these backward stretching exercises reduce your buttocks, hips, and
thighs while strengthening the muscles of
your lower back and abdomen. By restor-
ing the natural flexibility of your spine,
they also help prevent and correct
postural defects and relieve deep tension
throughout your back. In addition to the
exercises included here, the backward
stretching movements in Chapter 10 are
excellent for on - land or shallow water
practice. If you have a back problem,
check with your doctor before doing these
backward stretches.

Half Locust

—strengthens your abdominal muscles
—trims your hips and waist
Stand facing the wall an arm's length away with your hands close together holding at poolside.

Inhale, lifting your straight right leg back and up as you bend your elbows to bring your chin close to your hands. Keep your body straight without leaning to the left. (Figure 7-6)

Exhale, drawing your right knee toward your chest and your chin to your bent knee. (Figure 7-7)

Repeat three times with each leg.
On Land: Same

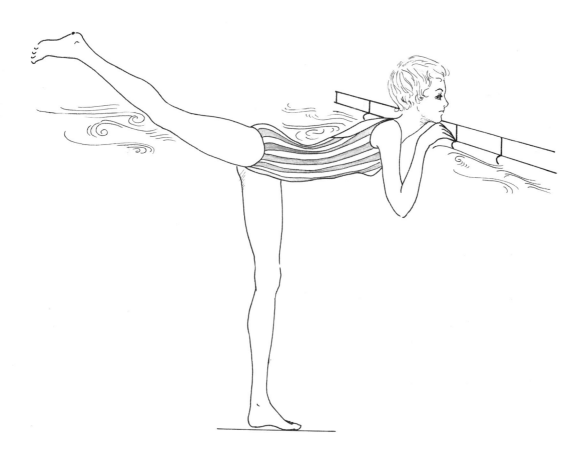

Figure 7-6

Figure 7-7

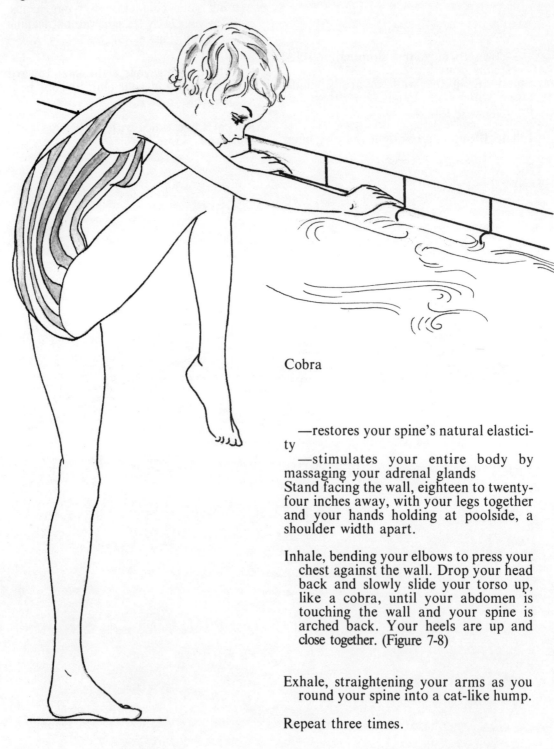

Cobra

—restores your spine's natural elasticity

—stimulates your entire body by massaging your adrenal glands

Stand facing the wall, eighteen to twenty-four inches away, with your legs together and your hands holding at poolside, a shoulder width apart.

Inhale, bending your elbows to press your chest against the wall. Drop your head back and slowly slide your torso up, like a cobra, until your abdomen is touching the wall and your spine is arched back. Your heels are up and close together. (Figure 7-8)

Exhale, straightening your arms as you round your spine into a cat-like hump.

Repeat three times.

Figure 7-8

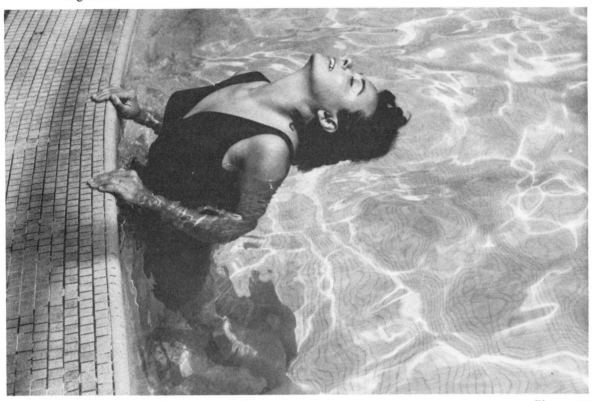

Figure 7-9

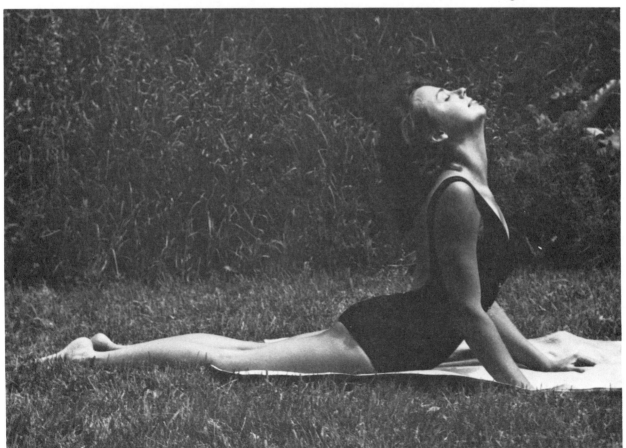

On Land: Lie face down on the floor with your hands, palms down, on the floor directly under your shoulders. Slowly curl your head and then your spine up and back toward your feet. Your pelvic area remains on the floor. (Figure 7-9) When you can no longer comfortably hold this position, slowly uncurl first your spine and then your head back to the floor.

Figure 7-10

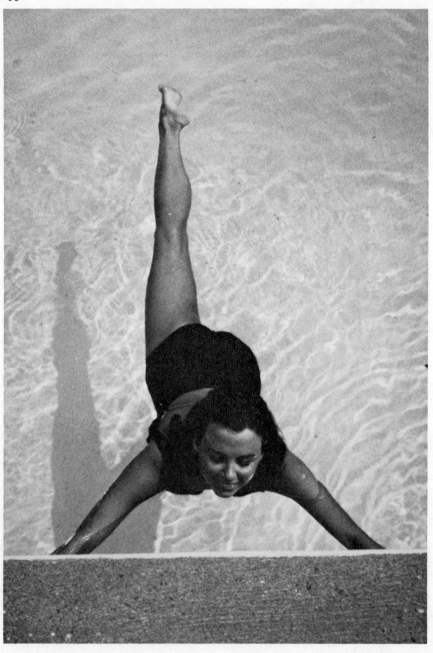

Elbow and Leg Lift

—trims your buttocks and thighs
—improves your posture
Stand away from but facing the wall so that you lean forward to stretch your arms into a wide V at poolside. Your legs are together with your heels down.

Inhale, raising your straight right leg back and up as you bring your shoulder blades together by raising your elbows several inches. Your shoulders are down and your hands still holding at poolside. (Figure 7-10)

Exhale, relaxing your arms and leg back to the starting position.

Repeat three times with each leg.
On Land: Same

Locust

—strengthens your lower back
Stand facing the wall, twenty - four to thirty inches away, with one hand holding at poolside, the other braced lower against the wall with fingers pointing down. Your legs remain straight and together throughout.
Inhale, raising your legs back and up. Feel your lower back muscles strengthening as you hold this position and your breath for a few seconds. (This is one of the few AQUAYOGA movements in which your breath is held.)

Exhale, lowering your legs again.

Repeat three times.
On Land: Lying face down with your chin

resting on the floor, clench your hands into fists and place them, thumbs down and palms facing each other, under your thighs. Inhale, raising your legs. Keep your chin on the floor. Hold that position and your breath. Exhale, lowering your legs to the floor.

Opposite Arm and Leg Bow

—restores natural flexibility to your thighs and spine
Face the wall with your feet together and your right hand holding at poolside. Bring your right foot back and clasp the front of it with your left hand.

Inhale, arching your back by pushing your foot out and up against your hand. Let your head drop back. (Figure 7-11)

Exhale, pressing your foot against your buttocks as you raise your head again.

Repeat three times with each leg.
On Land: Same

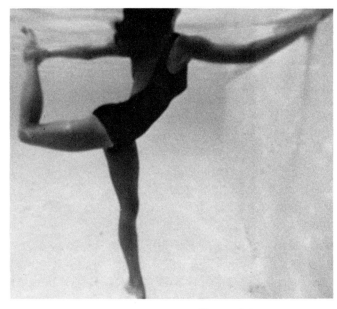

Figure 7-11

Figure 7-12

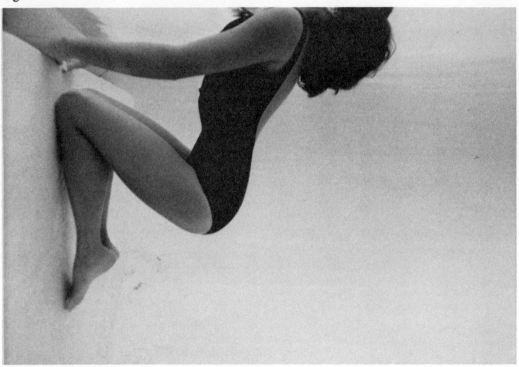

Figure 7-13

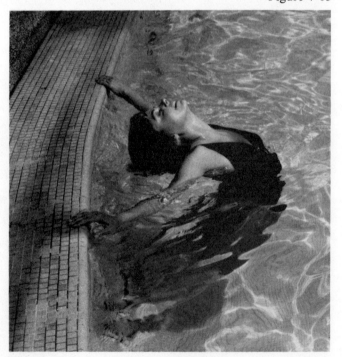

Back Stretch

—relieves tension in your shoulder
blade area
—maintains spinal flexibility
Face the wall with your hands, a shoulder
width apart, holding at poolside. Bend
your knees to your chest and place your
shins flat against the pool wall.
Straighten your elbows to push your torso away from the wall. (Figure 7-12)

Inhale, arching your back and lifting
your chest. (Figure 7-12)

Exhale, dropping your head back.

Remain in this arched position as you
move your head up and back again three
times.
On Land: Not practical

Cat

—relieves lower back pain
—improves your posture
Stand with your back to the wall and your hands holding at poolside. Your feet are close to the wall and slightly apart.

Inhale, pushing your hips forward away from the wall as your chest lifts up and your head drops back. Your heels are up. (Figure 7-13)

Exhale, rounding your back to the wall like a cat as you tighten your abdomen and rest your head on your chest.

Repeat three times.
On Land: Same

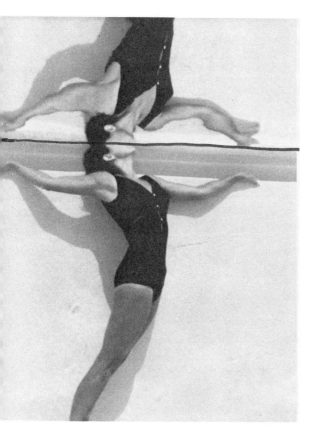

Boat

—strengthens your abdominal muscles and lower back
Stand with your back to the wall and your hands holding at poolside. Draw your knees up to your chest and then over to your left elbow with your left hip against the wall.

Inhale, stretching your legs straight behind with your toes on the pool floor and your back arched. Let your head drop back. Your left hip is still against the wall. (Figure 7-14)

Exhale, bending your knees first to your left and then over to your right elbow in order to repeat the stretch on the other side.

Repeat three times on each side.
On Land: Lie face down on the floor with your arms stretched overhead. Inhale, raising your straight legs, arms and head. Exhale, lowering them to the floor again.

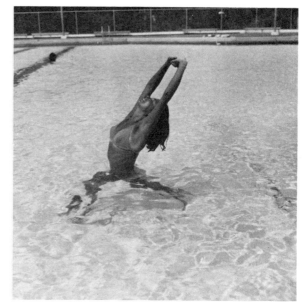

Figure 7-14   Figure 7-15

Backward Lunge

—stretches the muscles of your spine, abdomen and legs
—improves your posture
Stand stiff-kneed, away from poolside, with your right foot far in front of your left. With your hands forward, intertwine your fingers and raise your arms overhead with palms facing up.

Inhale, stretching your arms up even higher. (Figure 7-15)

Exhale, bending your right knee as you arch your back and stretch your arms and head backward. Tighten your abdominal muscles to prevent over arching of your spine.

Repeat three times with each leg forward.
On Land: Same

Figure 7-16

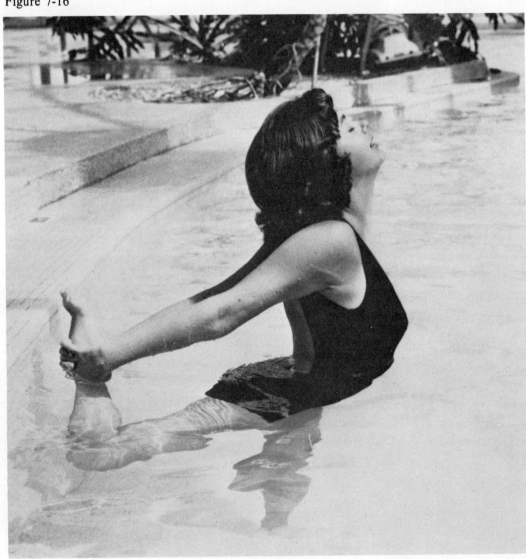

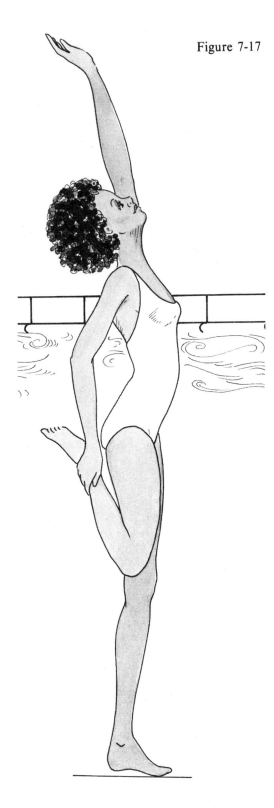

Figure 7-17   Bow

—trims your hips, buttocks and abdomen
—firms your bustline
Stand away from poolside with your feet together and your arms at your sides. Bring your right foot back and clasp the front of it with both hands.

Inhale, pressing your foot back and up against your hands so that your arms and leg are resisting one another. Let your head fall back to complete this delightful spinal stretch. Your body should look like an archer's bow, with your stretched arms and calf the string, and your head, trunk, and thigh, the curved strip of wood. (Figure 7-16)

Exhale, raising your head and pushing your heel against your buttocks.

Repeat three times with each leg.
If balance is a problem, hop gently on your standing foot or stand with your left side against the wall.
On Land: Lying face down on the floor, bend both knees and clasp the front of your ankles. Inhale, pushing your feet against your hands to raise your head, shoulders and thighs from the floor. Exhale, pushing your heels into your buttocks as you lower your head and shoulders again.

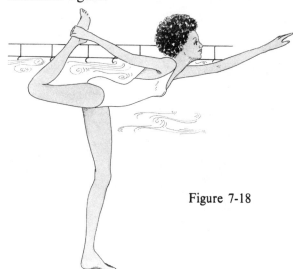

Figure 7-18

Arm and Leg Stretch

—relaxes deep tension in your spine and legs
—trims your hips and thighs
Stand away from poolside with your feet together and your arms at your sides. Bring your right foot back and clasp the front of it with your right hand. Press it against your buttocks.

Inhale, raising your left arm overhead and dropping your head back. (Figure 7-17)

Exhale, pushing your right foot up and out against your hand as you lean forward. Your head and left arm are up. (Figure 7-18)

Continue by inhaling to raise your left arm overhead with your head back as you press your right foot against your buttocks. Exhale by stretching your right leg and left arm into open arcs again. Repeat three times.
On Land: Same. Fix your gaze on something at eye level to help maintain balance.

Figure 7-19

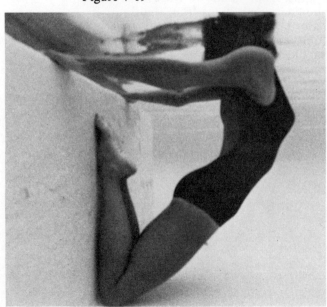

Swan

—prevents or corrects slumping shoulders
—maintains spinal flexibility
In waist - level water with your back to the wall, kneel on the pool floor with the tops of your feet against the wall and your toes pointing up. Your hands are holding at poolside.

Inhale, arching your back as you lift your chest forward away from the wall. Let your head drop back. (Fig. 7-19)

Exhale, returning your back and head to an upright position.

Repeat three times.
On Land: Lying face down on the floor with your hands on the floor directly under your shoulders, inhale, curling your head and spine back toward your feet. When you can go no higher, bend your knees to point your toes toward your head. Exhale, straightening your legs and uncurling your spine back to the floor again.

Twisting Stretching Exercises

The following exercises have a deeply relaxing effect on your nervous system. Your vertebral column is given a therapeutic twisting stretch that lengthens and tones your spinal muscles. Your lumbar muscles are particularly stretched and contracted, helping to reduce your waistline.

In addition to the exercises included here, the Twist in Chapter 10 is an excellent shallow water or on - land twisting movement.

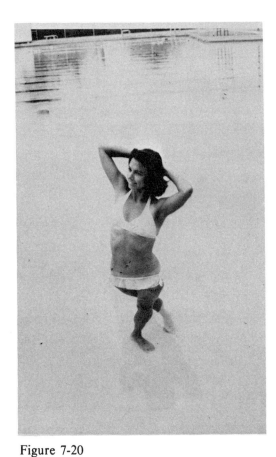

Figure 7-20

Zig-zag Walk

—trims your waistline
—provides a therapeutic twist to your spine
Stand away from poolside with your feet together and your hands clasped behind your head.
Step your right foot far over your left foot as you twist your torso to the left. Look back at your left elbow. (Figure 7-20)
From this position, step your left foot far over your right foot to twist to the other side.
Twist to alternate sides for one to two minutes. Maintain good posture with your pelvis tucked in and back upright.
On Land: Same

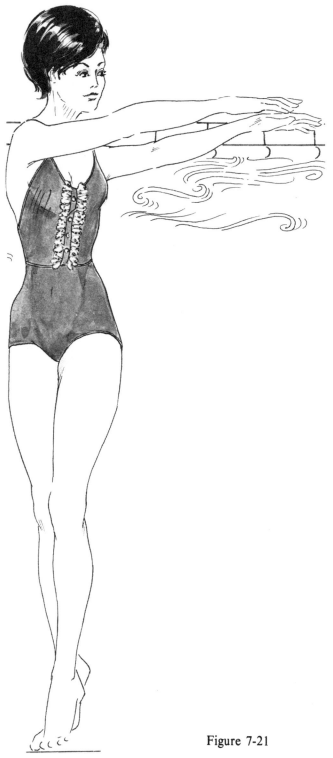

Figure 7-21

Toe Twist

—trims your waistline
—develops your balance
Stand on tiptoe away from poolside with
your arms stretched forward at shoulder
level, palms down.
Tiptoe forward on your left foot while
twisting both arms and torso to the left.
(Figure 7-21) Tiptoe forward on your right
foot and twist your arms and torso far
over to the right.
Continue in a rhythmic motion for one to
two minutes.
On Land: Out of the water, this becomes
a balancing position which strengthens
your ankles and feet. Stand on your toes
with your arms stretched forward at
shoulder level, palms down. Your feet remain stationary as you slowly twist your
arms and torso to the right. Hold this
position for a comfortable duration as
you keep your eyes on your fingertips to
develop balance and coordination. Then
slowly untwist your body to a forward
position again and relax before repeating
to the other side.

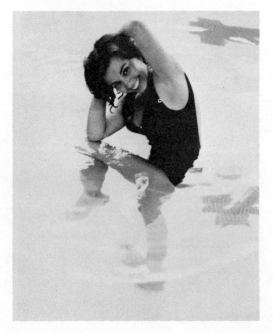

Figure 7-22

Elbow to Knee

—trims your waistline and abdomen
—relieves tension in your upper back
Stand away from poolside with your feet
together and your hands interlaced
behind your head.

Inhale, pressing your head and elbows
back. Notice the relief of tension in
your upper back. Your buttocks and
abdomen are tucked in tightly.

Exhale, raising your left knee and
twisting your torso to touch it with
your right elbow. (Figure 7-22)

Twist from side to side, alternating knees
and elbows, for one to two minutes.
On Land: Same

Horizontal Twist

—relieves tension in your upper back
—trims your upper arms
Stand away from poolside with your feet wide
apart and your right arm stretched forward,
your left arm stretched behind, and both palms
facing to the right. Your arms remain straight
and at shoulder level throughout.

Inhale, gliding your right arm back,
pushing the water away as if you were
doing the breast stroke, as your left
arm moves forward. Now both palms
are facing to the left.

Exhale, returning to the starting position
by breaststroking back with your left
hand and moving your right arm
forward.

Repeat six times.
On Land: Same

Crocodile Series

—trims your hips and abdomen
(1) Stand with your back to the wall and your hands holding at poolside. Cross your right ankle over your left foot and keep it crossed throughout.

Inhale, twisting your left hip against the wall and pointing your right hip forward. Press your right shoulder back against the wall. Concentrate on arching your middle back between your shoulder blades.

Exhale, twisting your right hip to the wall as you press your left shoulder back.

Repeat three times, and then reverse the direction of the twist by crossing your left foot over your right.
On Land: Lying on your back with your arms at shoulder level, palms down, cross your right ankle over your left foot and twist onto first your left hip and then your right hip. Your shoulders remain down throughout. Reverse by crossing your left ankle over your right foot and rolling onto first your right hip and then your left.

Figure 7-23

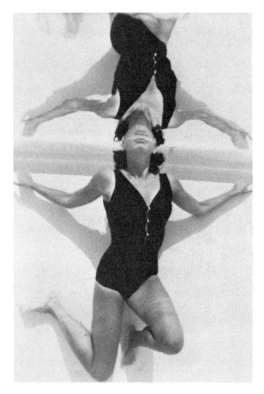

Figure 7-24

(2) Stand with your back to the wall and your hands holding at poolside. Place your right foot on the front of your left thigh with toes pointed down.

Inhale, twisting to the left to touch your right knee to the wall. Push back with your right shoulder and feel a delightful stretch in your spine. (Figure 7-23)

Exhale, gliding your knee over to the wall on your right while pushing back with your left shoulder.

Repeat three times with each leg.
On Land: Lying on your back with your arms at shoulder level, palms down, place your right foot on top of your left thigh and twist your knee to alternate sides. Your shoulders remain down throughout. Reverse.

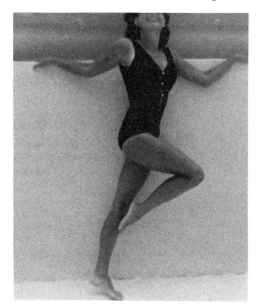

(3) Stand with your back to the wall and your hands holding at poolside. Bend your knees and place the soles of your feet on the wall twenty - four to thirty inches apart.

Inhale, bending your right knee toward your left foot with the sole of your right foot facing up. Your left knee is still pointing forward. (Figure 7-24)

Exhale, returning your knee to the starting position

Repeat three times with each knee.
On Land: Lying on your back with your

arms at shoulder level, palms down, bend your knees and place your feet on the floor, twenty - four to thirty inches apart. Bend alternate knees to the opposite foot.

(4) Stand with your back to the wall and your hands holding at poolside. Place the soles of both feet on the wall, twenty - four to thirty inches apart.

Inhale, pressing both knees to the wall on the left. (Figure 7-25)

Exhale, pressing both knees to the wall on the right. Enjoy the delightful stretch in your hips and thighs.

Figure 7-25

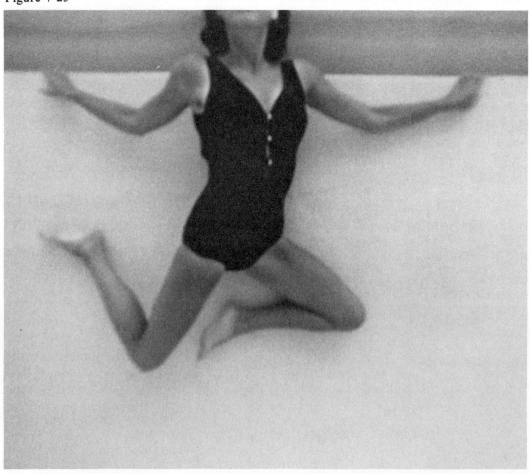

Standing Twist

—trims your waistline
Stand away from poolside in waist-level
water with your feet slightly more than a
shoulder width apart and your arms out-
stretched to the sides at shoulder level,
palms down.

Inhale, twisting your torso to the right.

Exhale, grasping the outside of your right
  knee with your left hand. Look up at
  your raised right hand. Reverse by inhaling to an upright position and
  repeating to the opposite side.

Repeat three times on each side.
On Land: Same

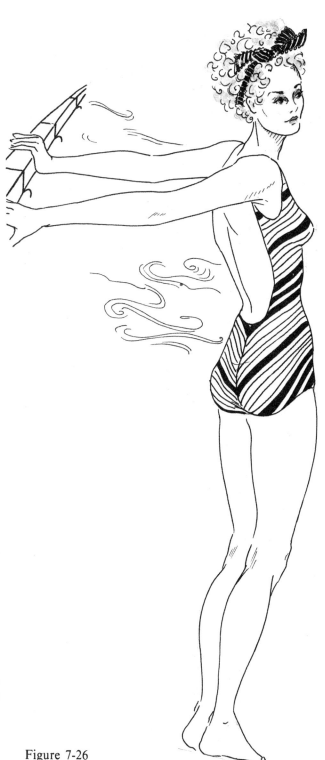

Arm Twist

—trims your arms and waistline
—firms your chest muscles
Stand with your left side away from the
wall so that you must lean slightly toward
the wall as you hold at poolside with your
left hand. Your feet are together and your
right arm is to the side at shoulder level,
palm facing back.

Inhale, watching your right hand as it
  glides back through the water to touch
  the wall behind you. (Figure 7-26)

Exhale, reversing your palm and returning your right arm forward and across to
  meet your left hand again.

Repeat three times with each arm.
On Land: Same

Figure 7-26

Figure 7-27

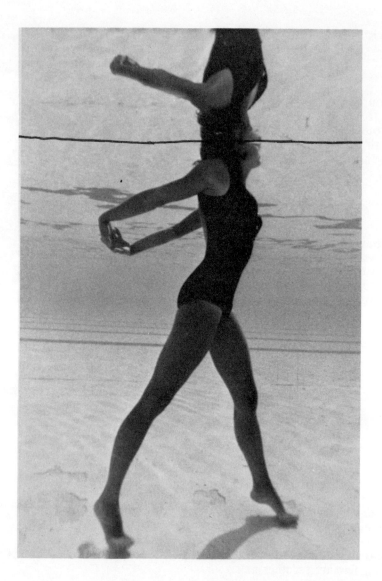

Chest Expansion Twist

—firms your chest muscles
—improves your posture
Stand away from poolside with your feet slightly more than a shoulder - width apart. Interlace your fingers behind your waist with your palms facing forward. Straighten your elbows and raise your arms high. Your back is straight with your abdomen and buttocks tucked in.

Inhale, keeping your arms high as you twist to the left and look over your left shoulder. (Figure 7-27)

Exhale, twisting to the right.

Repeat this tension-relieving sequence six times.
On Land: Same

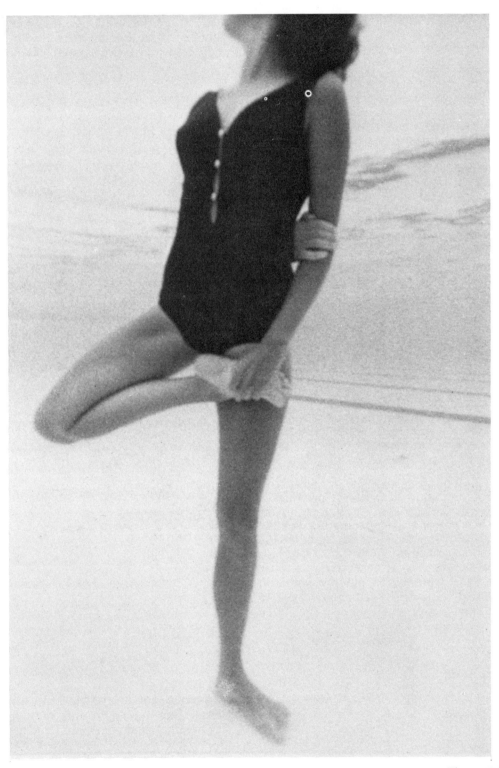

Figure 7-28

Half Lotus Twist

—maintains the flexibility of your ankles, knees, and hip joints
—relieves tension in your legs
Stand away from poolside with your feet together and your arms at your sides. Place the outside ankle of your right foot on top of your left thigh so that the bottom of your foot is facing forward. This is the Half-Lotus Position. If your ankle is not flexible enough to assume this position, place the sole of your right foot high on the inside of your left thigh with toes pointed down. Clasp your right foot with your left hand.
Slowly twist your right arm behind your lower back so that your torso and head twist back as well. Clasp your left elbow with your right hand. (Figure 7-28)
Repeat three times on each side.
On Land: Same. Fix your gaze on something at eye level to aid balance.

Sideward Stretching Exercises

The following exercises, in addition to reducing your waistline, provide a therapeutic sideward stretch to your spine, relaxing and strengthening the relatively weak side muscles. Holding the maximum sideward stretch for a comfortable duration is a particularly effective waistline trimmer. Avoid the common error of leaning forward as you bend to the side.

Side Bend

—trims your waistline
Stand with your left side an arm's length

away from the wall, feet together, and your left hand holding at poolside. Your right arm is overhead, palm out.

Inhale, stretching your right arm even higher.

Exhale, bending to the left. Keep your left arm straight and your right arm close to your head.

Repeat three times with each side.
On Land: Same

Hip Lift

—trims your waistline and hips
Stand facing the wall with your feet together and your hands, a shoulder width apart, holding at poolside.

Inhale, bending your torso sideways to the left. Keep a good tucked - in position as you feel a stretch down your right side. Your legs are straight.

Exhale, bending your torso sideways to the right.

Repeat three times.
On Land: Same

Overhead Stretch

—trims your thighs, hips and waistline
Stand with your right side to the wall, feet together, and your right hand holding at poolside. Your left arm is to the side at shoulder level, palm down.

Inhale, raising your straight left leg to the side toward your left hand, kneecap facing forward.

Exhale, gliding your leg down and across your right ankle as you stretch your left arm overhead, leaning to the right. (Figure 7-29)

Enjoy the good stretch in your left side. Repeat three times on each side.
On Land: Same

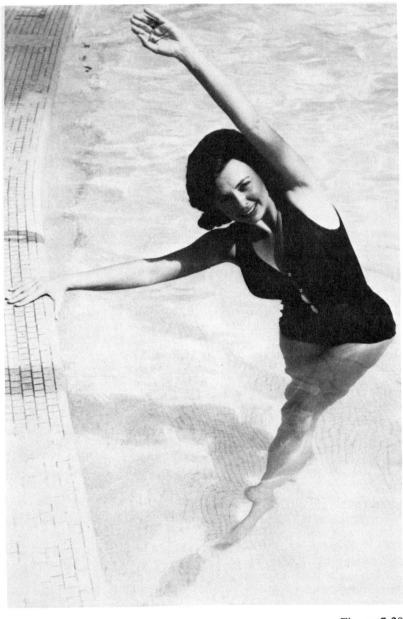

Figure 7-29

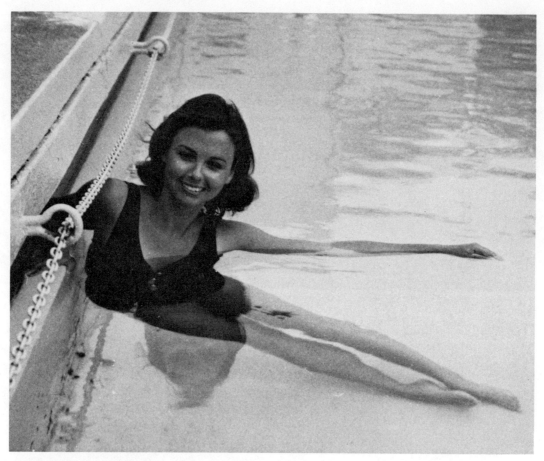

Figure 7-30

Hip to Wall

Elbow Side Stretch

—trims your hips and waistline
Stand with your right side an arm's
length away from the pool wall, your feet
together, and your right hand holding at
poolside.

Inhale, bending your right elbow to press
your right hip to the wall. (Figure 7-30)

Exhale, straightening your arm as you
return your hip to the starting position.
Repeat three times with each hip.
On Land: Same

—trims your waistline
Stand away from poolside in waist -
level water with one foot far in front of
the other and both knees bent.
Interlace your hands behind your head
with your elbows back.

Inhale, bending sideways to the right so
that your elbow is level with your
waist.

Exhale, bending to the opposite side.

Repeat three times.
On Land: Same

Triangle

—trims your waistline
Stand away from poolside in waist - level water with your feet a shoulder width apart and your arms at your sides. Your arms and legs remain straight throughout.

Inhale, raising both arms sideways to shoulder level, palms down.

Exhale, bending to the left to rest your left hand on the outside of your left knee. Keep your right arm against your right ear.

Reverse by inhaling to an upright position and exhaling to the other side. Repeat three times in each direction.
On Land: Same

Lunge and Stretch

—trims your waistline and hips
Stand facing the wall in a sideward lunge position with your right knee bent out to the side. Your right hand is holding at poolside.

Inhale, stretching your left arm overhead.

Exhale, bending sideways to the right. Keep your left arm at your left ear.

Repeat three times on each side.
On Land: Same

Chapter 8
Spot Reducing Exercises

The following exercises concentrate on trimming specific areas of your body, although many of them overlap to reduce other areas as well. Even though many of them are also excellent overall movements, be sure they are part of a more thorough program which systematically exercises your whole body.

Increasing the speed of these exercises will whittle away unwanted inches sooner. The faster you move, the more effort required of your muscles to work against the water's resistance and the sooner you will get results. Six repetitions of the exercises you choose is a good general guide, but you can begin with two or three and gradually work up to ten or twenty. Do a few stretching exercises afterward to eliminate any tension that may have built up. To keep warm in cool water or on chilly days, intersperse these brisk movements among the gentler stretching ones.

Shoulders, Chest and Arms

The exercises listed here have three main targets: (1) your upper back and shoulder muscles; (2) the network of

muscles that support your breasts; and (3) your upper arms. Many of these muscles are interdependent. Slumping upper back muscles prevent the important network of chest muscles and ligaments from properly supporting your breasts. Daily activities requiring only bent elbows cause your upper arm muscles to droop into sagging folds.

Many of the exercises here, with the effective aid of the water's resistance, help correct all these problems at once. Backward arm movements strengthen and tone your upper back, improve your posture and trim your upper arms. Forward arm movements strengthen your chest muscles. Arm circling limbers and shapes your shoulders as it firms your upper arms. By keeping your arms straight and your hands cupped like a scoop whenever possible in these exercises, the water's resistance is increased, and your upper arms are more efficiently reduced.

Shoulder Circling

—relieves tension in your shoulders and upper back
Stand away from poolside with one foot

far in front of the other. Bend your knees so that your shoulders remain submerged throughout the exercise. Your arms are relaxed at your side.

Draw a rectangle with your shoulders by bring them back, up, forward and down. As they move back and up, concentrate on your shoulder blades coming together in the back. As they move forward and down, round your back as if to separate your shoulder blades.

After three rotations, reverse the direction three times.

This is an excellent movement for relaxing between more strenuous exercises.

On Land: Same

Arm Rotation

—trims your upper arms

Stand away from poolside with one foot far in front of the other. Bend your knees so that your shoulders remain submerged throughout the exercise. Your straight arms are out to the sides at shoulder level with palms facing up. Keep your arms at shoulder level throughout.

Inhale, twisting your straight arms by facing your palms down and then behind.

Exhale, untwisting your arms by facing your palms forward and up.

Repeat twenty times. You may want to increase the speed of this upper arm - trimmer, making small vigorous circles without coordinated breathing.

Vary this movement by stretching your arms forward at shoulder level, palms up

and rotating your palms down and out to the sides.

On Land: Same

Pendulum Swing

—trims your upper arms
—relieves tension in your back

Stand away from poolside with one foot far in front of the other and both knees bent. Stretch your arms forward at shoulder level with palms down. Your arms remain straight throughout.

Inhale, swinging your arms down and back behind you.

Exhale, reversing your palms and pushing your arms down, forward and up to shoulder level again.

Repeat six times.

Vary the movement by beginning with one arm back and one forward and continually reversing their position.

On land: Same

Horizontal Arm Swing

—Tones the muscles of your upper back and chest

Stand away from poolside with one foot far in front of the other, knees bent. Stretch your arms out to the sides at shoulder level with palms facing back. Your legs remain stationary throughout.

Inhale, pushing the water away as you move your arms and head back. Think of bringing your shoulder blades together while keeping your buttocks and abdomen tucked in.

Exhale, with palms reversed, pulling your arms forward through the water and crossing them. Contract your abdomen. Either keep your arms straight or bend your elbows to hug yourself. Imagine bringing your shoulders together in front of you for a maximum expansion of your back.

Repeat four times.
Vary this movement by placing your fingertips on your shoulders with your elbows at shoulder level. Inhale, pressing your elbows and head back. Exhale, bringing your elbows together in the front with your chin resting on your chest.
On Land: same

Arc Swing

—tones your shoulder and chest muscles
Stand away from but facing the wall in waist - deep water so that you must lean forward from your hips to hold with your left hand at poolside. Stretch your right arm out to the side at shoulder level, palm down. Your arm remains straight throughout.
Swing your arm down; in front of, and across your body to the left in a motion parallel to the pool wall. Reverse your palm and swing your arm back to shoulder level.
Repeat six times with each arm.
On Land: Same

Arm Crossovers

—tones your shoulder and chest muscles
Stand away from poolside with your legs comfortably apart and your arms out to the sides at shoulder level, palms down. Keep your arms straight whenever possible.
Swing your arms down in front of your knees and cross them. Reverse your palms and swing your arms back to shoulder level. With palms facing down again, swing your arms behind your back and cross them. Face your palms up as you return your arms to shoulder level. Continue one to two minutes.
On Land: Same

Arm Circling

—trims your upper arms
Stand away from poolside with your feet comfortably apart and your arms at your sides, palms facing out.

Inhale, raising your arms forward as you bring your hands together back to back, palms facing out. Continue bringing your straight arms overhead.

Exhale, separating your hands as you lower your arms behind and down. Think of relaxing your shoulder blades as they gently move toward your spine. (It is this latter movement that is so effective in relieving and preventing tension in your upper back).

Repeat three times.

For a faster variation of this movement, spring up as you begin to circle your arms and land with both feet together on the pool floor as your arms circle back and down. Let your arms propel you out of the water with each upward movement. (Figure 8-1) Feel like a child exhuberantly splashing in the water as you continue to jump high and circle your arms for

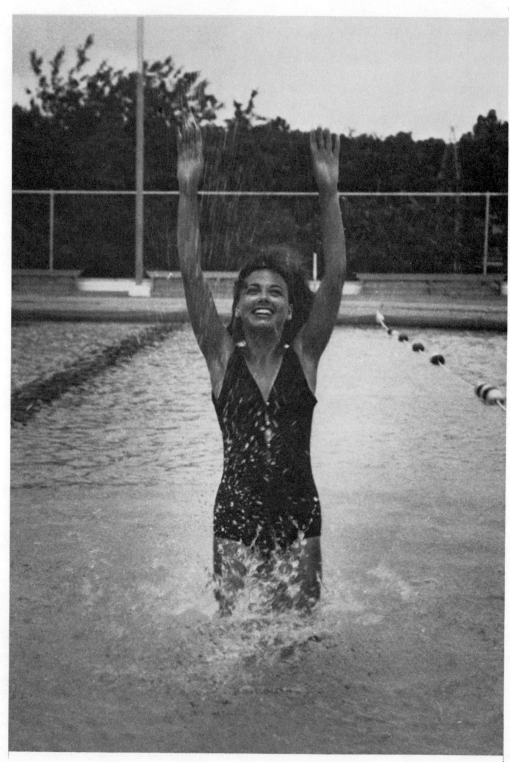

Figure 8-1

several minutes, reversing the rotation occasionally. This exercise is a marvelous warm - up for cold water days.
On Land: same

Elbow Rotation

—relieves tension in your upper back
Stand away from poolside with one foot far in front of the other and your knees bent. Your fingertips are on your shoulders.
Rotate alternate shoulders by drawing large circles with your elbows so that when your right elbow is pointing up, your left is pointing down.
Continue for one to two minutes, reversing the rotation occasionally.
On Land: Same

Backward Elbow Jump

—relieves tension in your upper back
—trims your shoulders and upper arms
Stand away from poolside with your feet together and your fingertips on your shoulders. Keep your elbows at shoulder level throughout.

Inhale, jumping backward with both feet together as you stretch your elbows and head back.

Exhale, jumping forward with both feet together as your elbows meet in front. Let your head drop forward and contract your abdomen.

Jump rhythmically back and forth for one to two minutes.
On Land: Not practical

Elbow Jump

—relieves tension in your upper back
—increases your circulation
Stand away from poolside with your feet together and your fingertips on your shoulders, elbows pointing down.
Spring high out of the water as you circle your elbows high. Land on the pool floor with your feet together as you complete the circle with your elbows pointing down again. Your fingertips remain on your shoulders throughout.
Continue for several minutes, reversing the rotation occasionally and springing higher as your strength increases.
On Land: Not practical

Arm Glide

—trims your waistline and upper arms
Stand away from poolside with your feet comfortably apart, your left hand on your hip and your right arm to the side at shoulder level with palm facing forward. Your right arm remains straight throughout.
Watch your right hand skim the surface of the water as you twist your arm and torso forward and over to the left. Keep your abdomen and buttocks tucked in tightly. Reverse your palm and twist your arm and torso far back to the right.
Continue this twisting stretch in a flowing motion, four times with each arm.
On Land: Same

Arm Figure Eights

—trims your upper arms

Stand away from poolside with one foot far in front of the other, knees bent.
With your arms out to the sides slightly below shoulder level, palms down, draw large horizontal figure eights. Your arms and hands remain submerged throughout.
Repeat six times.
On Land: Same

Stand away from poolside with your feet comfortably apart. Interlace your hands behind your back with both palms facing forward.

Inhale, dropping your head back as you straighten your elbows and lift your arms high. Resist the inclination to let your abdomen and buttocks protrude. Keep your back straight.

Chest Expansion Arm Lift

Exhale, lowering your arms slowly again as you return your head to the starting position.

—trims your upper arms
—relieves tension in your upper back

Repeat three times.
On Land: Same

Figure 8-2

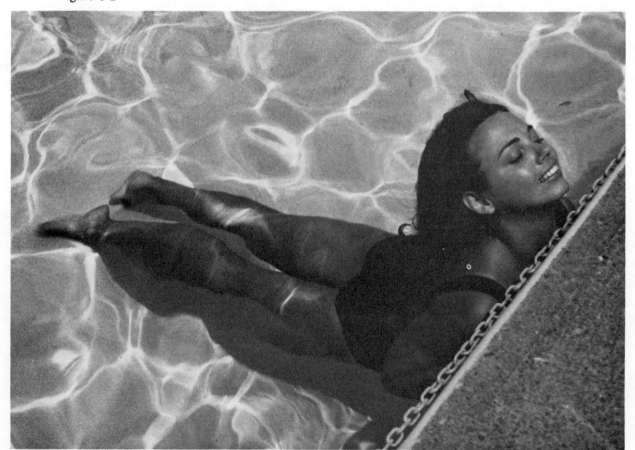

Push-up

Elbow and Foot Lunge

—strengthens your arms and chest muscles
Stand facing the wall two or three feet away so that you must lean forward to place your hands, shoulder-width apart, at poolside. Your lefgs are straight and together.

Inhale, bending your elbows to bring your chest to the wall. (Figure 8-2)

Exhale, straightening your arms as you return to the starting position.

Repeat six times.
On Land: Same

—tones your upper back and shoulder muscles
Stand away from poolside with your feet together and your fingertips on your shoulders.
Jump with your left foot and right elbow forward and your opposite leg and elbow behind. Both knees are bent. (Figure 8-3)
In one omotion, jump to reverse the position of your legs and elbows.
Continue for one to two minutes.
On Land: Not practical

Figure 8-4

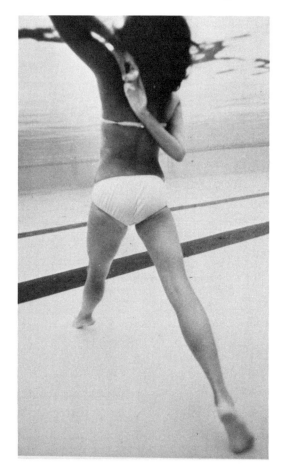

Figure 8-3

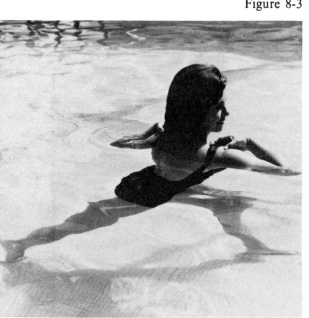

Backward Hand Clasp

—firms your upper arms
—prevents and corrects a slumping upper back
Stand away from poolside with your right foot far forward and your left foot behind. Bring your left hand behind your waist with your palm facing back. Join your hands together by reaching over your right shoulder with your right hand. (Figure 8-4) If your hands are far apart, try holding the ends of a bathing cap strap with either hand.

Inhale, dropping your head back with your right upper arm close to your right ear.

Exhale, returning your head to an upright position.

Repeat three times.
Advanced Variation: With your hands in the Backward Hand Clasp, gently pull your left hand up with your right hand; then pull your right hand down with your left hand. Your arms may move only several inches.
On Land: Same

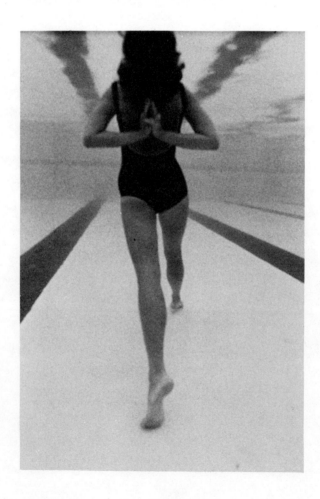

Figure 8-5

Prayer Position

—firms your upper arms
—maintains wrist flexibility
Stand away from poolside with one foot far in front of the other.
Behind your back hold your palms together with your fingers pointing down as if you were praying. With palms still together, point your fingers toward your lower back and then up toward your shoulders. Try to keep your palms together as you move your hands higher up your back. (Figure 8-5) Hold motionless for a comfortable duration before slowly lowering and relaxing your hands.

Repeat three times.
On Land: Same

Abdomen and Waistline

As times goes by, your internal abdominal structure and your stomach muscles tend to sag. This can become a serious problem because then your muscles no longer hold in place those internal organs that depend upon proper positioning to function well. It is encouraging to know that even though your abdomen and waistline are often the first to show added weight, they are also usually the first to respond to exercise. Any forward leg lifting in the water helps strengthen your abdomen. Any side bending of your torso and twisting of your upper back or hips will reduce the shape of your waistline. Maintaining good posture while exercising gives you an instantly slimmer look. By keeping your buttocks tucked under and your abdomen held in, you will whittle away your waistline and abdomen more quickly. In addition to the exercises in this chapter,

your waistline will respond to any of the twisting and sideward stretches in Chapter 7. The Abdominal Lift in Chapter 8 is also excellent for strengthening and trimming your abdomen.

Arm Lifts

—firms your abdomen and arms
Stand with your back leaning against the wall and your feet together. Your arms are at your sides, palms facing forward. Tighten your abdomen and press the small of your back against the wall. Maintain this tucked - in position throughout to firm your abdomen and improve your posture.

Inhale, lifting your arms forward, palms up, to shoulder level.

Exhale, raising your left leg forward as you reverse your palms and pull your arms down through the water to the wall.

Repeat with both arms and alternate legs for one to two minutes.
On Land: Same

Backward Arm and Leg Swing

—trims your waistline
—strengthens your lower back
Stand with your left side to the wall, feet together, with your left hand holding at poolside. Your right arm is overhead, palm facing forward.

Inhale, in one motion, stretching your right arm and head back as you raise your straight right leg behind you.

Exhale, pulling your arm forward, down and behind as you raise your right knee toward your chest. Bend your body forward slightly as if to put your chin on your knee.

Repeat three times on each side.
On Land: Same

Knee Raises

—trims your abdomen and hips
Stand with your back to the wall, your feet together, and your hands holding at poolside.
Raise your right knee to your chest. Swing it over to your left elbow, over to your right elbow, back to the center and down again.
Repeat three times with each knee.
Vary the movement by raising both knees up, swinging them to alternate sides, back to the center and down again.
On Land: Lying on your back with your arms at shoulder level, palms up, raise both knees up to your chest and over to alternate elbows.

Alternate Leg Raise

—stretches your leg muscles
—strengthens your abdominal muscles
Stand with your back to the wall, your feet together and your arms at your sides.

Inhale, raising your straight right leg and gently pulling it up by clasping your calf with both hands.

Exhale, releasing your hands and lowering your leg down through the water again.

Repeat three times with each leg.
On Land: Lying on your back with your straight right leg raised perpendicular to the floor, clasp your calf and gently pull your leg toward your face. Repeat with your other leg.

Leg Crossover

—strengthens your abdominal muscles
Stand with your back to the wall and your hands holding at poolside. Your legs remain straight and together throughout the exercise.

Inhale, raising your legs forward and high toward the surface of the water.

Exhale, swinging them over to touch your right hand at the wall.

Continue by inhaling as they return to the center and exhaling as they move to the other side. Repeat for one to two minutes.
On Land: Lie on your back with your arms stretched out at shoulder level, palms up. Raise your straight legs perpendicular to the floor. Keep them together as you lower them to alternate hands.

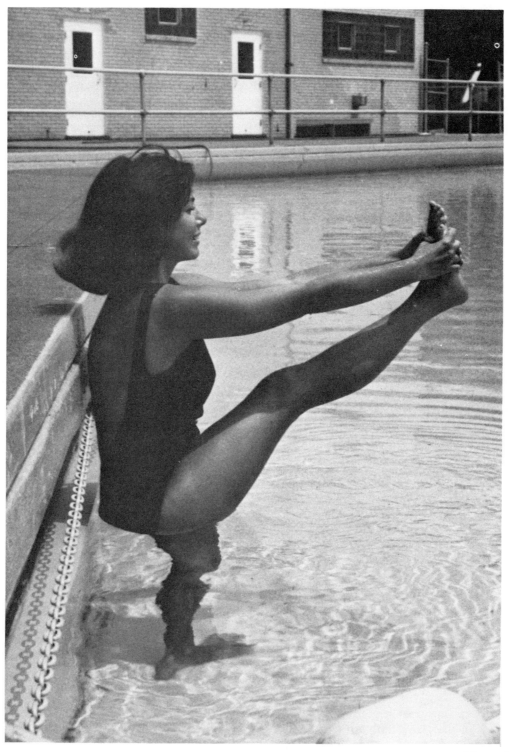

Figure 8-6

Leg Stretch

—trims and relaxes your legs

Stand with your back leaning against the wall and your feet together. Raise your right knee to your chest and clap the bottom of your foot with intertwined hands. It may be more comfortable for you to clasp your ankle or calf.

Inhale, straightening your leg by pushing your foot forward against your hands so that your leg is parallel to the pool floor. (Figure 8-6)

Exhale, returning your knee to your chest.

Repeat three times with each leg.

On Land: Lie on your back with your right knee at your chest and your hands intertwined around the bottom of your foot. Straighten your leg by pushing your foot upward against your hands. Repeat with your left leg.

Leg Lift

—strengthens your abdominal muscles
—trims your buttocks

Stand with your back to the wall, your feet together, and your hands holding at poolside. Try to keep the small of your back against the wall throughout. Your legs remain straight and together.

Inhale, raising your legs toward the surface of the water with your heels flexed.

Exhale, lowering your legs to the pool floor with your toes pointed.

Repeat six times.

On Land: Lying on your back with your hands under your buttocks, palms down, raise and lower your straight legs.

Wall Crawl

—stretches the muscles of your back for a deep relief of tension

Face the wall and hold at poolside with your hands a shoulder width apart. Place your feet close together high on the wall and gently straighten your knees.

Remaining in this position, inch sideways along the pool wall by stepping to the left with your left foot and left hand. Your right foot and hand follow after.

Continue inching to the left with alternate sets of hands and feet for one minute. Return by leading with your right hand and foot.

On Land: Not practical

Head to Knee Swing

—restores natural elasticity to your legs and spine

Face the wall and hold at poolside with your hands a shoulder width apart. Place your feet close together high on the wall with your knees bent.

Inhale, in one motion, straightening your knees and swinging your body to the right. Your feet stay in contact with the wall.

Exhale, returning to the center with your
knees bent.

Repeat by swinging to alternate sides in a
continuous fluid motion for one to two
minutes.
On Land: Not practical

Body Stretch

—firms your abdomen
Face the wall and hold at poolside with
your hands a shoulder width apart. Bend
your knees and place the soles of your
feet high on the wall slightly apart.

Inhale, vigorously kicking your straight
legs back behind you. Press your hands
against the wall and straighten your
elbows so that your body is parallel to
the pool floor.

Exhale, returning your feet to the wall
with your knees bent.

Repeat three times.
On Land: Not practical

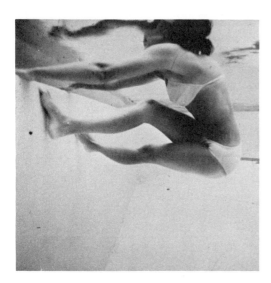

Figure 8-7

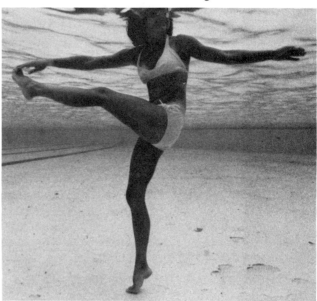

Figure 8-8

Wall Crossover

—trims your waistline
Face the wall and hold at poolside with
your hands a shoulder width apart. Place
your feet close together high on the wall.
Your arms and legs remain straight
throughout.
Alternately criss - cross one foot far over
the other so that you feel the action in
your waistline. (Figure 8-7)
Continue for several minutes.
On Land: Not practical

Figure 8-9

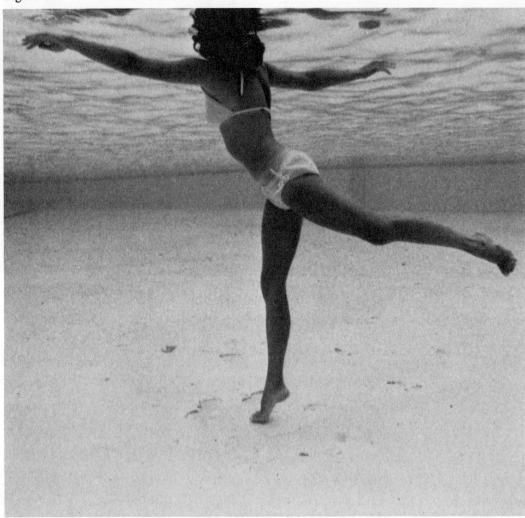

Alternate Toe Touch

—trims your abdomen, waistline and hips
Stand away from poolside with your feet comfortably apart and your arms to the sides at shoulder level, palms facing forward.

Inhale, raising your left leg forward and touch your left foot with your right hand. Stretch your left arm back and look over your left shoulder. (Figure 8-8)

Exhale, swinging your left leg backward as you twist your torso to the right with your left arm forward and your right arm back. (Figure 8-9)

Repeat six times on each side.
On Land: Same. Watch your balance!

Waistline Bounce

—firms your chest and upper arms
—prevents or corrects a rounded upper back
Stand away from poolside with your feet together and your arms stretched overhead, palms together.
Jump in place with both feet as you bend to one side and then the other, feeling a tremendous stretch on each side of your waist. (Figure 8-10)
Jump and stretch for one to two minutes.
On Land: Same sideward stretch but without jumping.

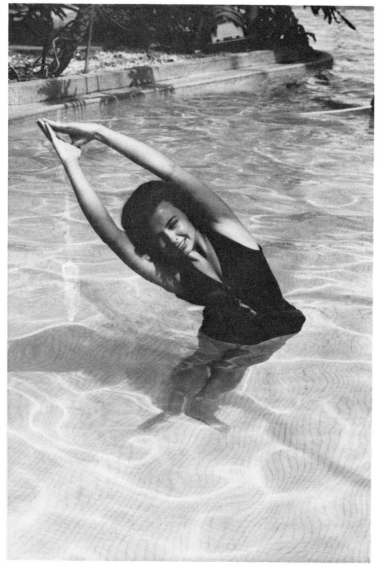

Figure 8-10

Figure 8-11

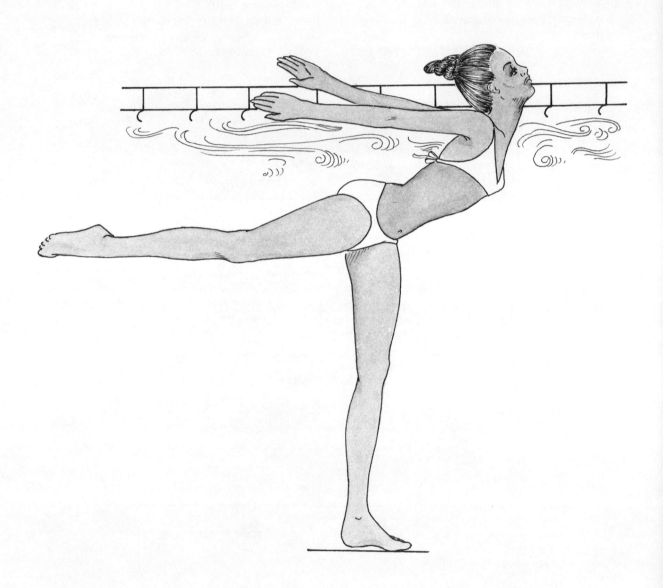

Figure 8-12

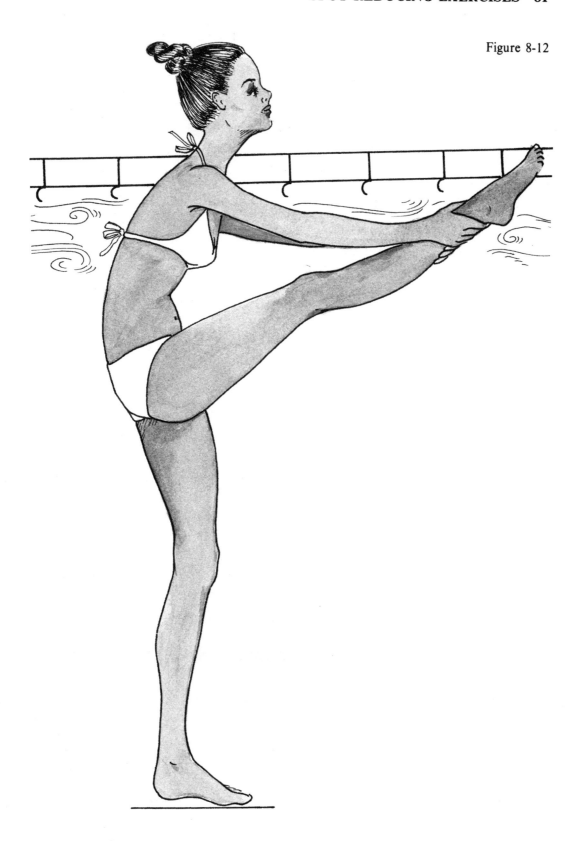

Backward Arm and Leg Stretch

—trims your buttocks and abdomen
Stand away from poolside with your feet
together and your arms stretched out to
the side at shoulder level, palms back.
Your legs are straight throughout.

Inhale, lifting your right leg behind as
you stretch your arms and head back.
Think of pulling your shoulder blades
together in the back. (Figure 8-11)

Exhale, raising your right leg forward
and up to grasp your ankle with both
hands. Swimmers can exhale under the
water, touching your head to your
knee. Otherwise, keep your head up.
(Figure 8-12)

Repeat three times with each leg.
On Land: Same

Dancing Twist

—trims your hips and waistline
Stand away from poolside with your feet
twelve to eighteen inches apart and your
knees bent and together with toes pointing in. Your straight arms are forward,
slightly below shoulder level, with both
palms facing to the right. Bend forward
slightly and tuck in your abdomen. Now
you are ready for an interesting variation
of the popular dance of the fifties—the
twist.

Inhale, gliding your arms far to the right

while pointing your right hip forward.
Let your right heel come up. (Figure
8-13) Be aware of your hip muscles
working as you feel the stretch in your
waist.

Exhale, reversing your palms and pulling
your arms to the left as you point your
left hip forward. Let your left heel
come up.

Twist for one to two minutes.
On Land: Same

Figure 8-13

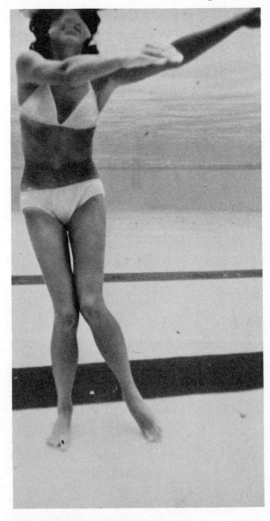

Figure 8-14

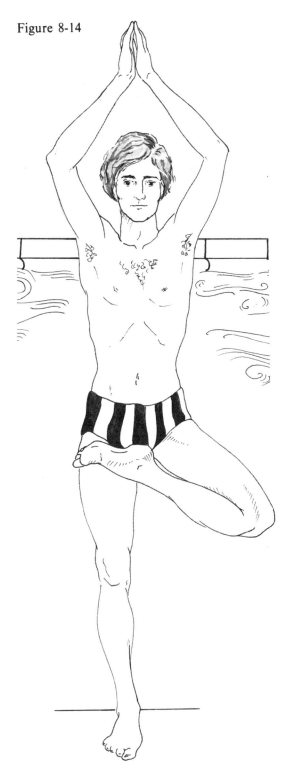

Tree

—trims your waistline
—develops balance

Stand away from poolside with your feet together and your arms at your sides. Slowly place the top of your left foot on your right thigh so that your knee is pointing out to the side and the bottom of your foot is facing up. (Never force your foot into this half-lotus position. With patience and performance of other exercises, flexibility will eventually come.) If you are not flexible enough yet, place your foot high on the inside of your right thigh.

Slowly stretch your arms overhead with your palms together as if praying. (Figure 8-14) If balance is a problem, either bounce gently on your standing foot whenever necessary or stand sideways against the pool wall. Hold for four to six deep breaths.

Relax and repeat two more times.

On Land: Same. Fix your gaze on something at eye level to help maintain balance.

Figure 8-15

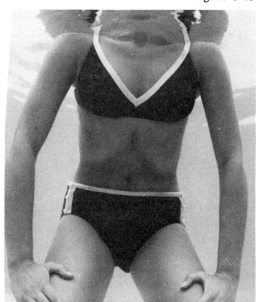

Abdominal Lift

—firms your abdomen
—prevents constipation
Stand away from poolside with your feet comfortably apart. Bend your knees slightly and place your hands firmly on your thighs with your fingers pointing inward.
Inhale deeply and then exhale completely. Without inhaling again, pull your abdominal muscles back to your spine and up under your ribs. (Figure 8-15) Hold this position motionless for five to ten seconds. Then inhale deeply, and, relaxing your abdomen, exhale completely and pull your abdominal muscles back and up again.
Stand with three repetitions and gradually increase to ten.
With practice, especially in the water where your body feels so much lighter, this deep contracting and raising becomes easier as your abdominal muscles become stronger. It is most effective when done on an empty stomach.
On Land: Same

Hip Swing

—trims your waistline and hips
In water over your head, face the wall with your hands a shoulder width apart, holding the ladder or at poolside. Your legs are straight down and together; your abdomen and buttocks are tucked in. As if to draw an arc parallel to the pool wall, swing your straight legs sideways to the right, back to the center, and over to the left. Feel the action in your waistline as you fishtail against the resistance of the water.

Continue for several minutes in a swinging motion.
On Land: Not practical

Hips, buttocks and Thighs

Your hips, buttocks and thighs are three of nature's favorite fat depositories and are often the most difficult areas to rid of excess weight. Because the water demands extra effort of your muscles, the following exercises are often more effective than on - land ones to help trim these hard - to - reach spots. Sideward leg lifts dissolve fat on the sides of your hips and the outside of your rights. Backward leg lifts trim your buttocks and thighs as they strengthen your lower back. Especially effective in the water are inward leg movements from a spread - apart position since your inner thigh muscles are forced to work harder than they ordinarily do out of the water.
Remaining active can prevent the hip and thigh spread that often comes with age. Walking, jogging and squatting, either in or out of the water, help maintain firm buttocks, thighs and hips. Swimming and bicycling are also excellent reducers of these areas. If you must lead a sedentary life, double your efforts with the exercises in this chapter as well as the Locust and Half - Locust in Chapter 7.

Leg Crisscross

—trims your hips
Stand with your back to the wall, your

feet together, and your hands holding at poolside.

With stiff knees, crisscross your legs by stepping your right foot far over your left foot and standing on it. Then step your left foot over your right in the same manner.

Repeat in a continuous motion for one to two minutes.

On Land: Same

Rapid Leg Lifts

—trims your hips, buttocks and thighs

Stand facing the wall with your feet together and your hands, a shoulder width apart, holding at poolside. Your legs remain straight throughout.

Rapidly kick your right leg backward four times. Then swing it sideways to the right four times.

Repeat six times with each leg.

On Land: Same

Side Arm and Leg Swing

—trims your hips and waistline

Stand with your left side an arm's length away from the wall, feet together, and your left hand holding at poolside. Your legs remain straight throughout.

Inhale, in one motion, lifting your right leg to the side with kneecap facing up as you stretch your right arm overhead.

Exhale, swinging your leg and arm, like a pendulum, down and across in front of your body.

Repeat six times on each side.

On Land: Same

Alternate Leg Circling

—trims your hips and thighs

Stand with your left side to the wall, feet together, and your left hand holding at poolside. Your right arm is out to the side at shoulder level, palm down.

Inhale, raising your right leg forward and then high to the side.

Exhale, circling your leg back behind and down to the pool floor again.

Repeat six times with each leg.

On Land: Same

Leg Figure Eight

—trims your hips and thighs

Stand with your left side to the pool wall, feet together, and your left hand holding at poolside. Your right arm is to the side at shoulder level, palm down.

Raise your right leg sideways, kneecap facing up, and draw a large horizontal figure eight with your leg. Your leg remains straight throughout.

This same movement can be done with your back to the wall.

Repeat six times with each leg.

On Land: Same

Figure 8-16

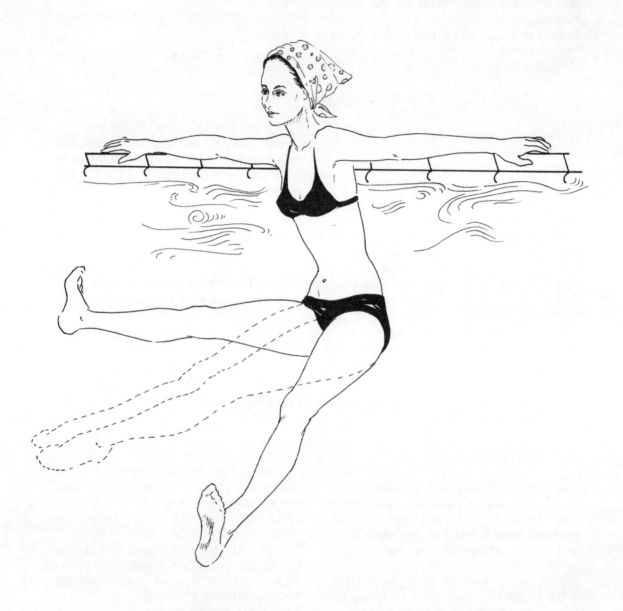

Forward Arm and Leg Swing

—firms your abdomen and arms
Stand with your left side to the wall, feet together, with your left hand holding at poolside. Your right arm is at your side with palm facing back. Your legs remain straight throughout.

Inhale, raising your right leg forward with your heel flexed as you push your right arm back.

Exhale, reversing the position of your arm and leg by swinging your leg down and behind and your arm forward and overhead.

Repeat six times on each side.
On Land: Same

V Stretch

—trims your abdomen, inner thighs, and hips
Stand with your back to the wall and your arms and hands holding at poolside. Let your straight legs float forward and up. Keep the small of your back against the wall for extra strengthening of your pelvic girdle.

Inhale, flexing your heels with toes pointed up, as you stretch your legs apart to make a wide V. (Figure 8-16)

Exhale, pointing your toes, ballerina style, as you close your legs.

Repeat ten times.
Vary this movement by keeping your feet pointed either in toward one another or out to the side throughout.
On Land: Lying on your back with your hands, palms down, under your buttocks, raise your legs to a perpendicular position. Stretch them apart with your heels flexed and close them with your toes pointed.

Foot Figure Eight

—restores natural flexibility to your ankles and calves
Stand with your back to the wall and your arms and hands holding at poolside. Let your legs float forward and up and spread them apart into a wide V.
Move only your ankles as you draw horizontal figure eights with your feet.
Repeat ten times.
On Land: Lying on your back with your hands, palms down, under your buttocks, raise your legs to a perpendicular position. Spread them apart into a wide V and rotate your ankles to draw horizontal figure eights with your feet.

Leg Circling

—trims your hips and thighs
Stand with your back to the wall and your arms and hands holding at poolside. Let your leg float forward and up and spread them apart into a wide V.
Draw large ovals with your legs by mov-

Figure 8-17

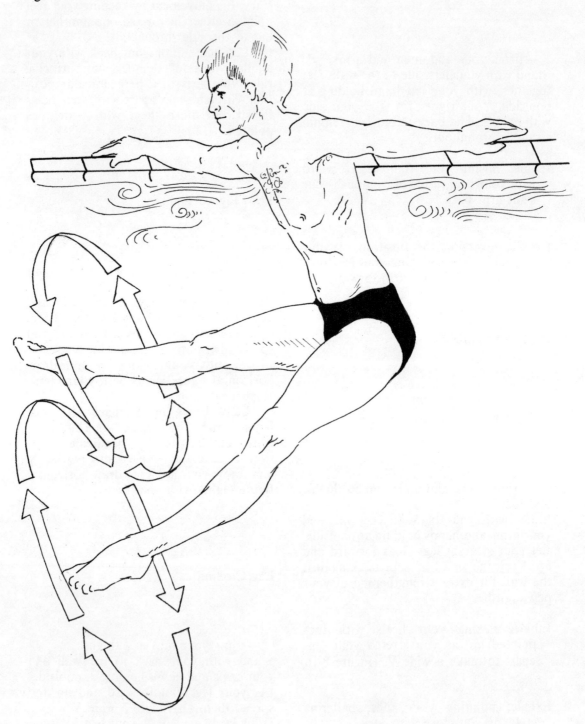

ing them both up, in, down, and out. (Figure 8-17)

Repeat six times and then reverse the direction six times.

Leg circling can also be done in a prone position with one hand at poolside and the other lower and flat against the wall with fingers pointing down.

On Land: Lie on your back with your hands, palms down, under your buttocks. Raise your legs to a perpendicular position and, with your feet apart, circle your legs both in, down, out, and up.

Side Leg Raise

—reduces your hips and thighs
—increases the flexibility of your hip joints

Stand away from poolside with your feet together and your arms to the sides at shoulder level, palms down.

Inhale, lifting your right leg sideways toward your right hand with your toes and kneecap pointing forward. Enjoy using those often neglected hip muscles again.

Exhale, lowering your leg to the pool floor.

Raise and lower your left leg in the same manner and continue with alternate legs for one to two minutes.

Vary this movement for a greater inner thigh stretch by pointing your toes to the side, kneecap facing up, as you raise your leg.

On Land: Same

Hip Rotator

—increases the flexibility of your hip joints

Stand facing the wall an arm's length away, with your feet together and both hands holding at poolside. Hook your left foot behind your right calf.

Swing your left knee out to the side and forward again as you feel the action in your lower back.

Repeat twelve times with each knee.

On Land: Same

Spread Leg Stretch

—stretches your inner thigh muscles
—reduces your hips

Face the wall and hold at poolside with your hands close together. Place your feet far apart high on the wall and gently straighten your knees. (Figure 8-18) If the wall of your pool has no ledge or gutter, hold the bars of the pool ladder with your feet apart on the wall. Gently bouncing in this position is a good preparation for the next exercise.

Inhale, gliding your right hip to the right as you bend your right knee outward.

Exhale, gliding to the left and bending your left knee.

Repeat in a continuous motion for one to two minutes.

Advanced Variation: Remaining in this spread leg position, walk down and back up the pool wall in four to six short steps for a good inner thigh trimmer.

On Land: Not practical

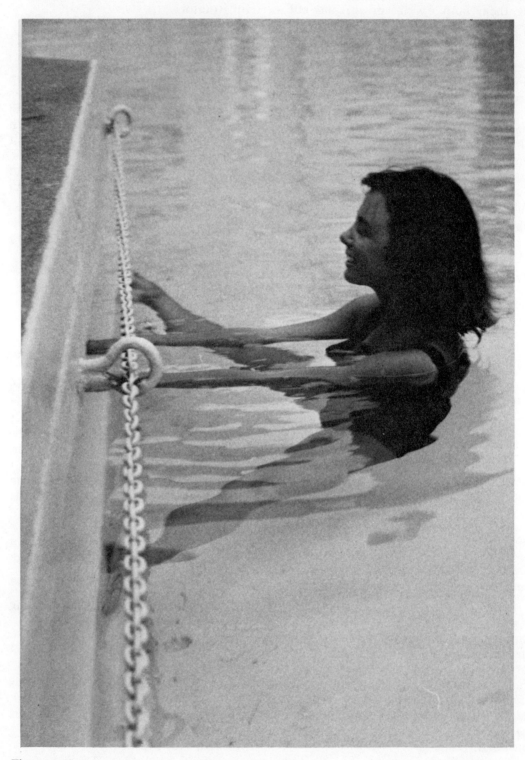

Figure 8-18

Wall Bounce

—trims your hips and thighs
Face the wall with hands, a shoulder width apart, holding at poolside. Place your feet close together high on the wall with your knees bent toward your chest. Bounce as you place your feet far apart high on the wall. Spring back to the bent - knee position in the center again. Repeat this bouncing stretch six times.
On Land: Not practical

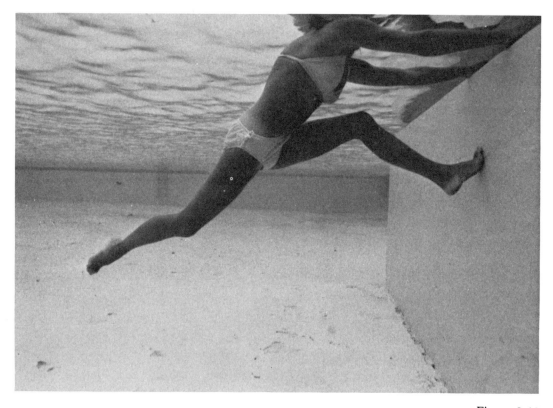

Figure 8-19

Figure 8-20

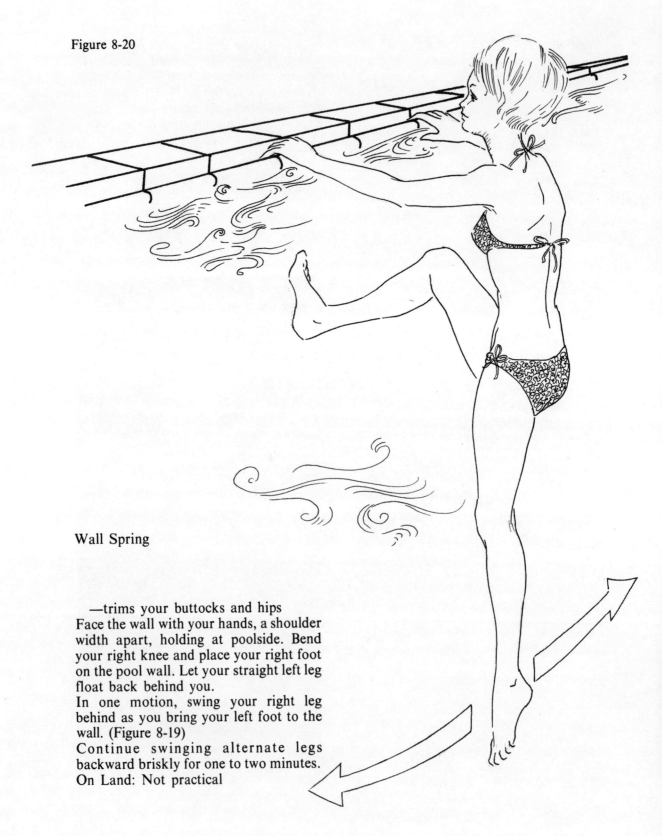

Wall Spring

—trims your buttocks and hips
Face the wall with your hands, a shoulder
width apart, holding at poolside. Bend
your right knee and place your right foot
on the pool wall. Let your straight left leg
float back behind you.
In one motion, swing your right leg
behind as you bring your left foot to the
wall. (Figure 8-19)
Continue swinging alternate legs
backward briskly for one to two minutes.
On Land: Not practical

Pendulum Leg Swing

—trims your hips and thighs
Face the wall with hands, a shoulder width apart, holding at poolside. Bend your right knee and place your right foot high up on the wall. Let your straight left leg float up behind you. Throughout the exercise, keep your arms and back straight and your left knee facing the pool wall.

Inhale, swinging your left leg sideways to the left. (Figure 8-20)

Exhale, swinging it sideways to the right.

Continue swinging your leg back and forth, pendulum style, in a motion parallel to the pool wall. Repeat six times with each leg.
On Land: Not practical

Figure 8-21

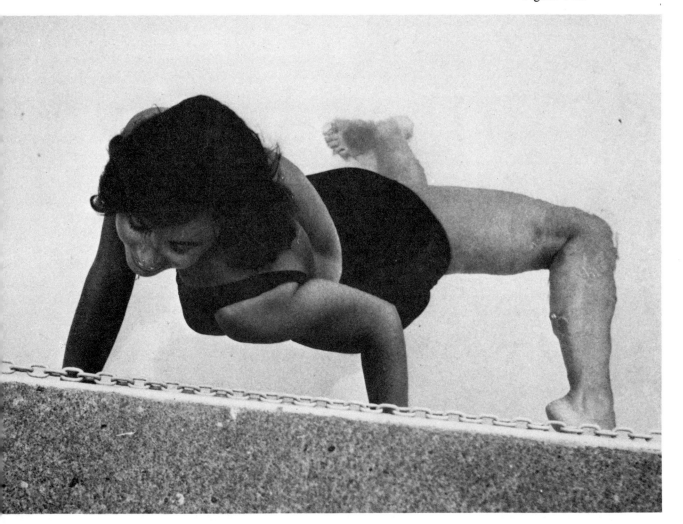

Bent Knee Lift

—trims your hips and waistline
Stand facing the wall with your hands far apart holding at poolside. Raise your right bent knee out to the side and then lift your right foot back behind so that your calf is parallel to the surface of the water. Keep your knee bent throughout. Leaning forward and keeping your foot high, glide it backward and across to touch the wall on your left side. (Figure 8-21) Return your knee along the same path to touch the wall on your right. Repeat four times with each leg.
On Land: Same

Bent Knee Balance

—trims your hips, waistline and abdomen
Stand away from poolside with your feet together and your arms at your sides. Raise your right knee high toward your chest and then point it to the left with your toes pointed. Raise your right arm overhead and bend your left arm behind your waist.

Inhale, straightening your right leg high to the right side with your knee cap facing up as you reverse the position of your arms.

Exhale, returning your arms and knee to the starting position.
Reverse so that your left knee is up and your left arm is overhead. Repeat three times with each side.

If balance is a problem, try the same sequence standing sideways to the wall with your left hand holding at poolside when your right leg is moving and vice versa.

On Land: Same

Wrists, Hands, and Fingers

Your hands often reflect your true mood. Relaxed, limber hands impart a feeling of serenity. Nail - picked, cuticle - bitten hands reveal tension and anxiety. How easy it is to recognize the nervous person who wrings his hands, anxiously taps his fingers, or fidgets with pen, hair, or glasses.
These exercises alternately tense and relax your hands and fingers to eliminate tension and increase flexibility. They can easily be done in a matter of minutes either in the bath or pool where the resistance of the water encourages extra muscular effort. Wherever you decide to do them, relax in any comfortable position and bend your elbows so your fingers are pointing forward and your palms are facing down. Repeat each exercise six times.
The skin of your hands has even fewer oil cells than that of your face, so apply a generous amount of cream after exercising in the water.

Thumb Stretch

Cross your thumbs over to touch the bottom of your small fingers. Return them to the starting position.

Thumb Circling

Draw wide circles with your thumbs, rotating them three times in each direction.

Finger Stretch

Beginning with your forefingers, alternately bend each finger down toward your wrists and back up again.

Hand Tenser

Spread your fingers and thumbs wide apart and tense them. Hold for a count of five and then relax them into loose fists.

Wrist Bend

Keeping your arms still, bend at your wrists to raise and lower your hands. Vary the movement by making fists instead of pointing your fingers.

Wrist Side Stretch

Moving only from your wrists with your arms still, point your hands in toward one another and then out to the sides. Vary the movement by making fists instead of pointing your fingers.

Wrist Rotation

Moving only from your wrists with your arms still, draw large circles with your hands. Vary the movement by making fists instead of pointing your fingers.

Finger Fan

With your hands in loose fists, turn your palms up as you spread your fingers far apart. Return them to loose fists.

Finger Flick

Beginning with your thumbs, quickly flick each finger up through the water as if to push a bug away.

Wrist Flick

With your fingers loose and relaxed, flick your wrists in a rapid upward motion six times.

The Knees

Your knees probably receive less attention than any other part of your body when exercising, yet it is important to keep them flexible and trim. The water makes it easier for you to move your knees in all possible ways more completely than on land. Try the following exercises both in and out of the water to see the difference.

Two types of knee exercises are included here: (1) knee movements to provide a therapeutic limbering of your knee joints and, (2) slapping your knees together to provide the friction necessary to reduce this hard - to - trim area. In addition to them, simly sitting with your knees bent outward in a cross - legged position is another effective exercise which loosens and relaxes your knee joints.

Knee Slap

—trims your knees
Stand with your back to the wall and your arms and hands holding at poolside. Bend your knees to your chest and slap them together.
Repeat this slapping motion twenty times.

On Land: Lying on your back with your knees bent and your feet flat on the floor, slap your knees together.

Charleston

—trims your knees and inner thighs
Stand away from poolside on tip - toe with your feet twelve to eighteen inches apart and your knees bent. Cross your hands in front of you and rest them on opposite knees.
Quickly do the Charleston by swishing your knees far out and gently slapping them together as you alternately uncross and cross your hands.
Continue for one to two minutes.
On Land: Same

Knee Bend

—reduces and limbers your knees
Stand facing the wall with your feet together and your hands holding at poolside.

Inhale, coming high up on your toes.

Exhale, bending your knees out to the sides as if to sit. Pull your buttocks together and in as you tighten your abdomen.

Repeat ten times.
This movement can be made progressively harder by doing it in shallower water.
On Land: Same

Can - Can

—trims your knees
—maintains knee flexibility
Stand with your back leaning against the wall. Raise your left knee and hold under your thigh with both hands.
Without moving your thigh, draw big circles with your foot, first in one direction, then in the other.
Circle twelve times with each leg.
On Land: Same

Ankles, Feet, and Toes

Maintaining flexibility and good circulation in your ankles, feet, and toes keeps them healthy and trim. Flexible toes add a bounce to your walk. Healthy feet are a source of relaxation rather than a source of tension and fatigue.

The following movements will provide the necessary exercise for your feet in a matter of minutes. They can be done as directed in the bath, the pool, or on land. If your feet are especially inflexible, the warm water of the tub is the best place to begin these exercises. To do them in the bath, sit with your legs extended in front of you and your arms resting comfortably on the sides of the tub. When doing them in the pool, stand with your back against the wall, your arms and hands holding at poolside and your legs floating forward and up. Your legs should remain straight throughout. Repeat each exercise six times.
Foot cramps are an indication of poor muscle tone. If they are a problem for you, continue the exercises cautiously. The cramps will lessen as your muscles become healthier.
The Foot Variations in Chapter 6 and the Backward Bend in Chapter 10 are good

additional foot exercises. Walking barefoot, especially in grass and sand, is also an excellent foot strengthener.

Heel Flex

Flex your heels, pointing your toes toward your chest; then point your toes forward.

Foot Side Stretch

Point your toes sideways to the left and then to the right, moving just your ankles, with your legs as still as possible.

Ankle Rotation

Begin to draw a wide circle with your feet by flexing your heels, toes pointed up, and moving them sideways to the left. Finish half the circle by pointing your toes down, ballet style. Continue to the right and up to the flexed position again. Reverse the rotation.

Toe Bend

Flex your heels so that your toes are pointing up. Your feet remain flexed; only your toes move. Curl your toes under, point them up again and then point them toward your knees.

your knees. Feel the muscles in the bottom of your feet strengthening.

Curled Toes Stretch

Toe Fan

With your legs stiff - kneed and slightly apart, curl your toes under as if to pick up something with them. Your toes remain curled throughout. Point your feet in toward one another and then up toward

Spread your toes apart sideways and close them up again by bending in the little toe first and trying to close each toe in succession up to your big toe.

Chapter 9
For Swimmers Only

Floating Exercises

These stretches are for those who can float both with face up and face down. In order to float well, it is important to keep your body straight. Your buttocks and abdomen should be tucked in tightly, your chest held high and your shoulders relaxed and back. If your legs sink, tuck your buttocks and abdomen in tightly again and raise your legs toward the surface. To stay afloat, always keep extra air in your lungs. Limit your exhalation so that some of your breath is retained as you immediately inhale again. Bending your wrists to raise your hands above the water's surface whenever your arms are overhead will also increase your buoyancy.

If exercising while floating is new to you, your first attempts may be awkward. Rather than floating free at first, you may prefer holding onto a kickboard or the pool's ledge for support. With some patience, you will develop an ease in doing these effective stretches.

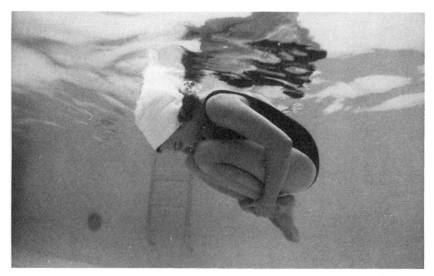

Figure 9-1

Child's Pose

Arm and Leg Lift

—relieves lower backache and strain
Float face down and hug your knees to
your chest.
Tuck your chin between your knees and
exhale slowly through your nose and
mouth. Feel a gentle stretch in your lower
back as you allow your body to drift
naturally. (Figure 9-1)
Repeat three times.
On Land: Two variations are possible: (1)
Lie on your back with your knees pressed
to your chest and your chin between your
knees; (2) From a kneeling position, sit
on your heels and bend forward to rest
your forehead on the floor with your
arms back alongside your body, palms
facing up.

—trims your arms and legs
—strengthens your lower back
Float face down in the water with your
arms stretched overhead, a shoulder
width apart, your straight legs together
and your toes pointed.
Exhale through your nose and mouth as
you lift your right leg and left arm high.
Lower and lift your alternate arm and
leg.
Repeat six times.
On Land: Lie face down on the floor with
your arms stretched overhead, and alternately raise your opposite arm and leg.

Figure 9-2

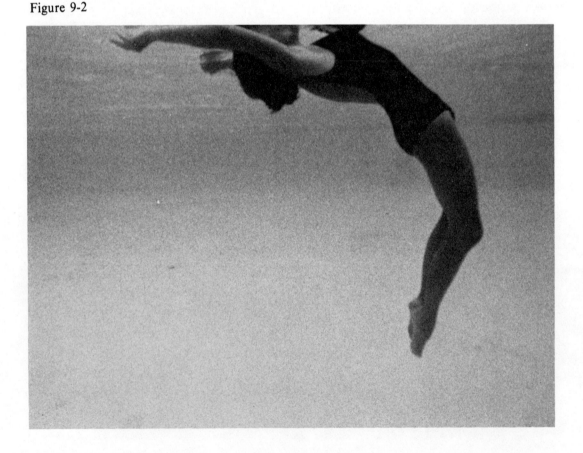

Boat   Crocodile Series

—trims your buttocks and thighs
—strengthens your lower back
Float on your back with your arms
overhead, a shoulder width apart, your
straight legs together, and your toes
pointed.

Inhale, arching your lower back as you
    stretch your straight legs backward
    toward the pool floor. (Figure 9-2)

Exhale slightly, drawing your bent knees
    up to the surface of the water as if you
    were sitting.

Repeat three times.
Vary this movement by floating face
down with your arms stretched overhead,
your straight legs together and your toes
pointed. In one motion, raise your arms,
head and straight legs.
On Land: Lie face down with your arms
stretched overhead and raise your arms,
head, and legs up. Lower them to the
floor again.

—trims your waistline and abdomen.
For all three rolling stretches, begin by
floating on your back with your arms
stretched overhead, a shoulder width
apart, your straight legs together and
your toes pointed.

(1) Cross your right ankle over your left
    foot. With your shoulders stationary,
    roll onto your left hip and arch your
    back, especially through your shoulder
    blade area. Return to the center and
    stretch your spine in the opposite
    direction by reversing the position of
    your legs and rolling onto your right
    hip.

Repeat three times to each side.
On Land: Same

(2) With your shoulders stationary, roll
    onto your right hip and slowly bend
    your left knee to place your left foot on
    your right thigh. (Figure 9-3) Relax to
    a back - floating position as you
    straighten your left leg.

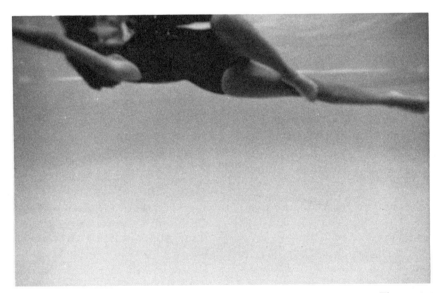

Figure 9-3

Repeat three times to each side.
On Land: Same

(3) With your shoulders stationary, roll onto your left hip. Bend both knees to the left so that your left foot is on your right knee. Relax on your back as you straighten your legs.

Repeat three times to each side.
On Land: Same

Side Stretch

—relieves tension throughout your entire body
Float on your back with your arms overhead, a shoulder width apart, your straight legs together and your toes pointed.
Stretch your right arm farther overhead as you stretch your right foot down. Feel the stretch in your hips.
Repeat three times on each side.
Vary the movement by stretching opposite arm and leg; then stretch both arms and both legs at once.
On Land: Lying on your back with your arms overhead, stretch back with your arms and down with your feet.

Hands to Shoulders

—prevents and corrects a rounded back
Float on your back with your arms at your sides, palms toward your body. Your legs are straight and together with toes pointed.
Keeping your elbows in, bend them to raise your hands sideways to your shoulders, palms facing out, in a modified

back stroke. Slowly return your hands to your sides.
Repeat ten times.
On Land: Not practical

V Arm and Leg Stretch

—trims your thighs and waistline
Float on your back with your arms at your sides and your legs together. Your arms and legs remain straight throughout.

Inhale, opening your legs and stretching your arms overhead. Your arms and legs are both forming a wide V.

Exhale slightly, closing your legs again as you press your arms to your sides.

Repeat three times.
Vary the movement by floating face down as you open and close your arms and legs.
On Land: Not practical

Scissors Kick

—trims your hips, thighs, and lower legs
—strengthens your lower back
Float on your right side with your right arm overhead, your left hand, palm down, in front of your chest and your heels flexed. Scissors kick rapidly back and forth.
Repeat six times. Relax by floating on your back and then repeat to the other side.
On Land: Lie on your right side with your right arm stretched overhead and your left hand on the floor in front of you. Lift your straight legs and scissors kick with a back and forth motion.

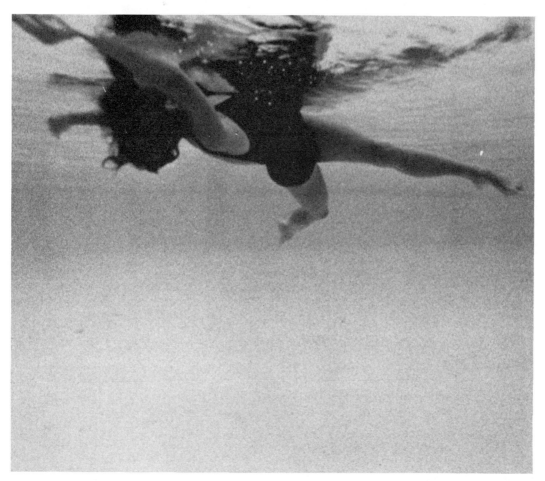

Figure 9-4

Scissors Turn

—trims your hips, thighs, and lower legs
—strengthens your lower back
Float on your back with your arms overhead, a shoulder width apart, your straight legs together and your toes pointed.
With your shoulders stationary, roll onto your right hip and scissors kick rapidly back and forth. (Figure 9-4)

Repeat six times on each side.
On Land: Not practical

Figure 9-5

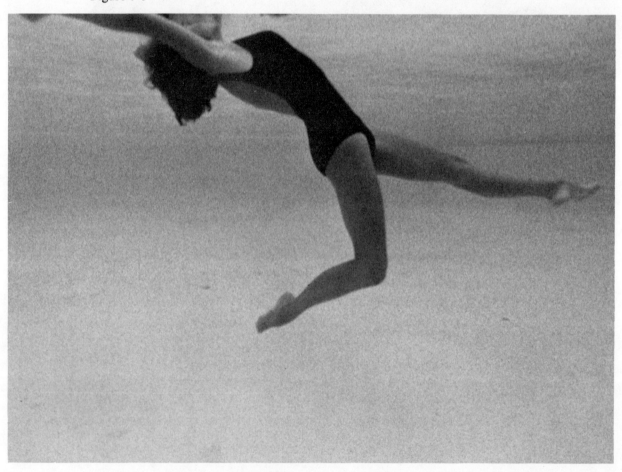

Knee Bend

—trims your thighs and buttocks
Float on your back with your arms
overhead, a shoulder width apart, your
straight legs together and your toes
pointed. Maintain a tucked - in position.

Inhale, bending your right knee to bring
your right foot down and back to meet
your buttocks. (Figure 9-5)

Exhale slightly, straightening your leg
again.

Repeat with alternate legs and then with
both legs together for one to two minutes.
On Land: Not practical

Underwater Exercises

When doing the following stretches,
always inhale out of the water and exhale
through your nose (and mouth if desired)
as you submerge. Hold each position for
a comfortable duration as you let your
body drift freely through the water.

Figure 9-6

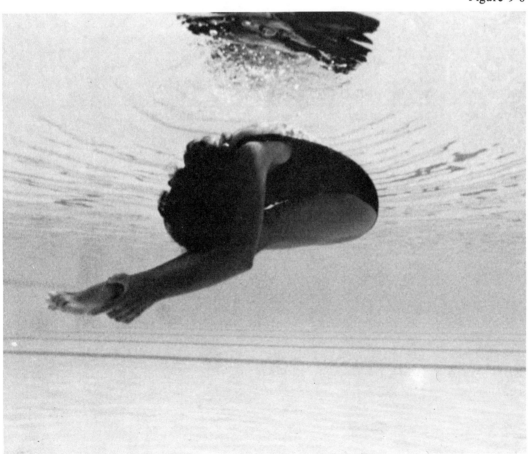

Head to Knee

—trims your abdomen
—stretches your entire spine
Stand away from poolside with your feet together and your arms at your sides. Exhale through your nose and mouth as you bend down to grasp your calves,

ankles, or feet, depending on your flexibility. Aim your forehead toward your knees. Allow your body to drift naturally. (Figure 9-6)

Repeat three times.
On Land: Sit with your legs together straight in front of you. Aim your head toward your knees as you reach forward to clasp whatever part of your legs you can.

Figure 9-7

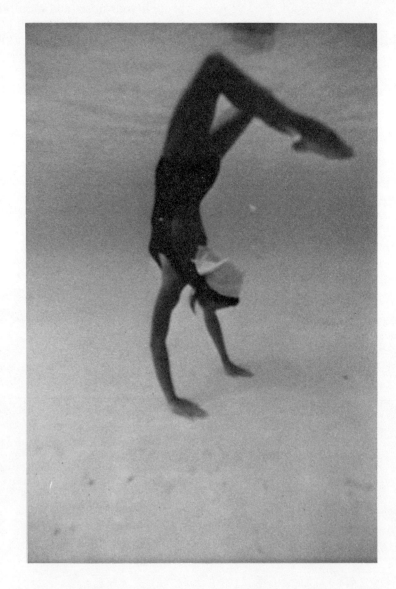

Backward Somersault

—provides a tension - relieving spinal stretch
—improves upper back posture
From a floating position on your back, exhale through your nose and mouth as you stretch your head and torso backward and under the water until you are facing the pool floor. Hold that arched position with the sides of your feet together, your knees apart, and your head back. Moving your arms in dog - paddle fashion or placing your hands on the pool floor helps maintain this backward stretching posture. (Figure 9-7) After a comfortable duration, continue to an upright position.

Repeat three times.
On Land: Not practical

Figure 9-8

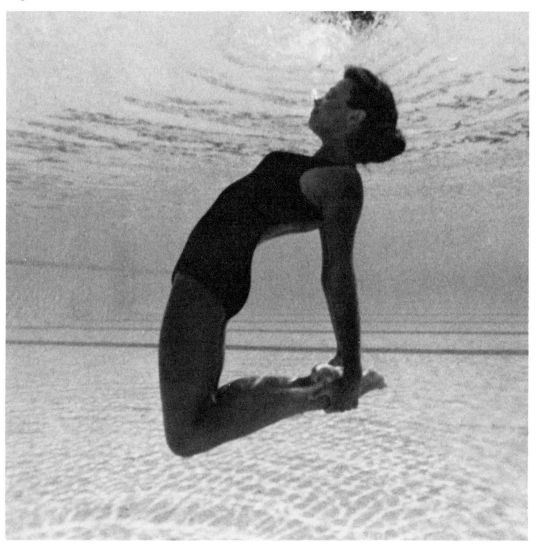

Bow

—provides a therapeutic backward stretch to your spine
—trims your thighs
From a floating position on your back, bend your feet behind you so that your hands can clasp your ankles. Push your feet against your hands to arch your back as you slowly submerge, exhaling through your nose. Your head remains forward throughout. Allow your body to drift naturally. (Figure 9-8) After a comfort-able duration, return to an upright position.

Repeat three times.
For a more intensive stretch of your front thigh muscles, press your feet against your buttocks instead of out against your hands.
On Land: Lying in a prone position, bend your feet back and clasp the front of them with your hands. With the sides of your feet together and your knees apart, push your feet against your hands to raise your head, shoulders, and thighs from the floor. Lower your body and relax.

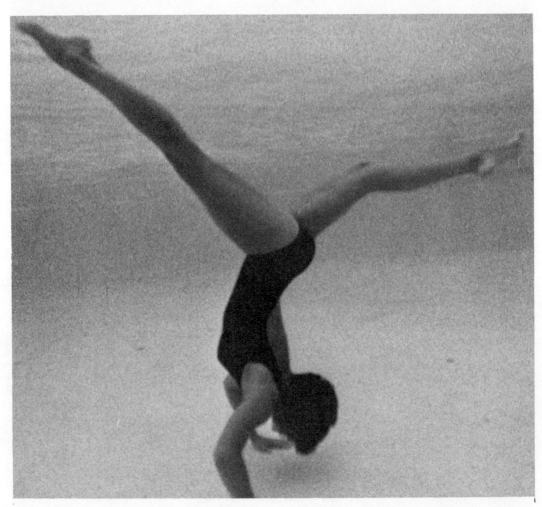

Figure 9-9

Headstand Split

—trims your thighs and buttocks
—provides a therapeutic stretch in your lower back

Stand away from poolside with your feet together and your arms at your sides.

Exhale through your nose and mouth as you bend forward, placing your hands on the pool floor and raising your legs overhead. Split your legs with one foot forward and the other back. (Figure 9-9) If balance is a problem, walk on your hands on the pool floor.

Repeat three times.

On Land: Balancing in the headstand on your forearms, hands, and head as explained in Chapter 1, split your legs with one forward and the other back.

Chapter 10

Exercises for the Bath or Wading Pool

All of the following exercises can be done as directed out of the water. But whenever possible, let the buoyancy and resistance of the water enhance these movements. The warm water in the bath or wading pool will also soothe and relax your muscles, helping to keep them limber.

Let your mood be your guide to how much you do. After a harried day, eliminate the strain in your face and body with the gentle Lion and the eye and neck exercises. Then recline with a folded towel behind your neck and do the Deep Relaxation Exercise from Chapter 2. If you are more energetic, limber up with several alternate leg raises. Then choose one or two exercises from the forward, backward, and twisting movements. (Side stretching is too awkward in the confining space of the tub.) Be sure to have a non - skid rubber bath mat on the tub floor to prevent slipping. By repeating each exercise three to six times, the entire series can be done in fifteen to twenty minutes. Your bath or shallow water routine can also include the exercises for your hands and feet in Chapter 8.

Leg Raise
—strengthens your abdomen

—Trims and relaxes your leg muscles
Sit with your legs together straight in front of you. Lean back slightly and stretch your arms forward, palms down.

Inhale, raising your straight right leg high.

Exhale, lowering it again.

Repeat three times with each leg.
Advanced Variation: Raise both legs together.

Leg Raise with Towel

—trims your legs and abdomen
Sit with your legs straight in front of you. Hold the ends of a towel and loop it around the bottom of your left foot. Your leg remains straight throughout.

Inhale, pulling the towel to raise your leg high. Keep your heel flexed. (Figure 10-1)

Exhale, lowering your leg into the water
again.

Repeat three times with each leg.

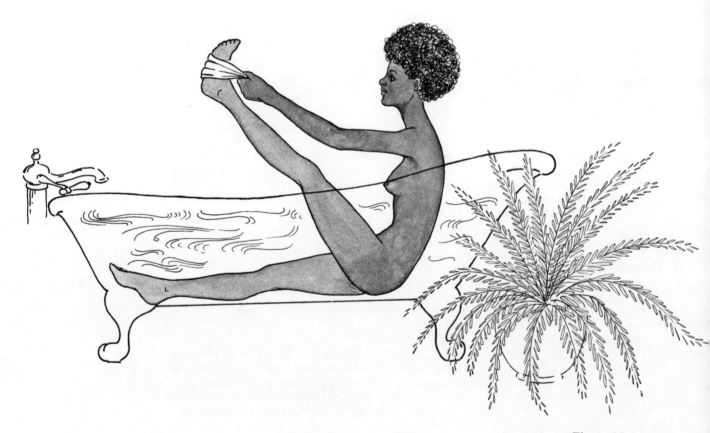

Figure 10-1

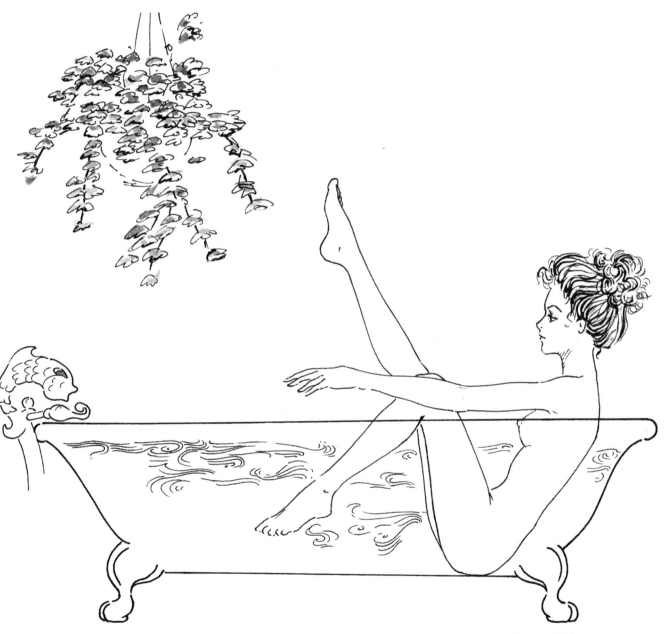

Figure 10-2

Alternate Leg Raise

—strengthens your abdomen
—trims and relaxes your leg muscles
Sit with your knees bent and your feet on
the floor. Lean back slightly and stretch
your arms forward, a shoulder width
apart, for balance. Raise your feet to

bring both knees to your chest.

Inhale, straightening your right leg vertically. (Figure 10-2)

Exhale, bending your right knee as you
straighten your left leg up.

Repeating in a continuous motion for one
to two minutes.

Figure 10-3

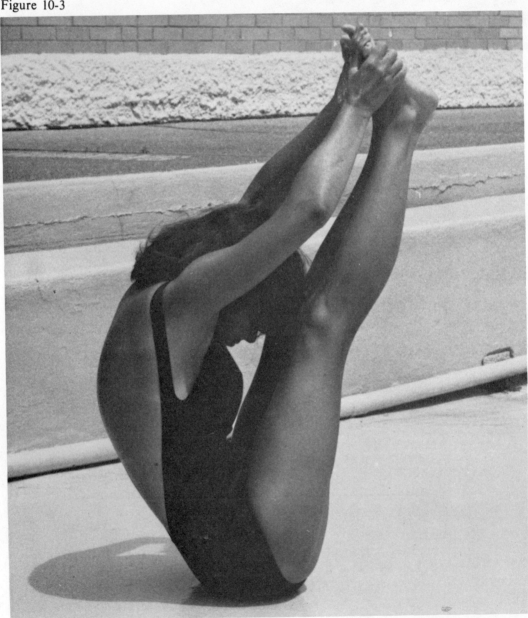

Advanced Variation (The Angle Pose): With your knees to your chest, grasp your feet and straighten both legs up vertically toward your forehead. (Figure 10-3)

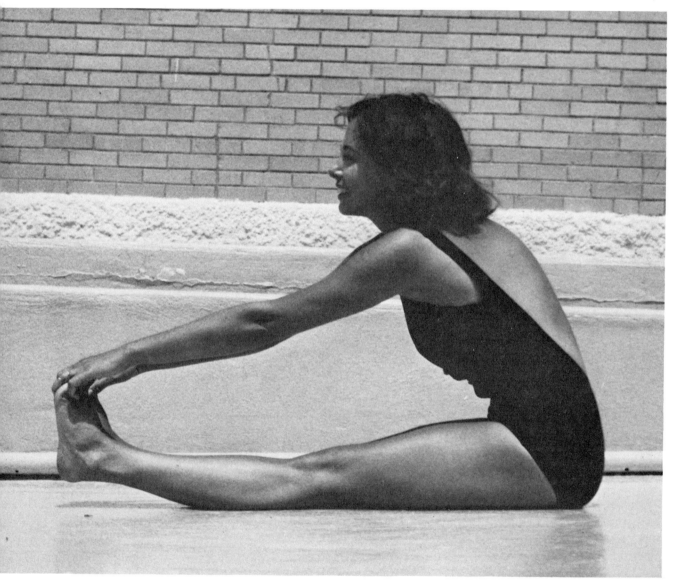

Figure 10-4

Leg Stretch

—trims and relaxes your leg muscles
Sit with your legs together straight in
front of you. If flexibility allows, grasp
the toes of both feet with your hands.
Otherwise, hold your ankles.

Inhale, pulling your toes or ankles up to
    raise your heels an inch or two from
    the floor. Your calves remain down.
    (Figure 10-4)

Exhale, lowering your heels.

Repeat three times.

Archer

—reduces your hips
—limbers your hip joints
Sit with your legs straight in front of you.
Place your left foot on your right thigh.
Hold your right toes or ankle with your
left hand.
Grasp the toes of your left foot with your
right hand and raise them toward your
right ear. (Figure 10-5)
Repeat three times on each side.

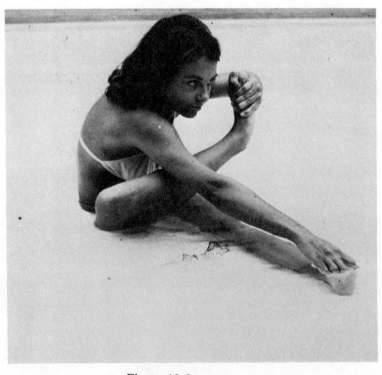

Figure 10-5

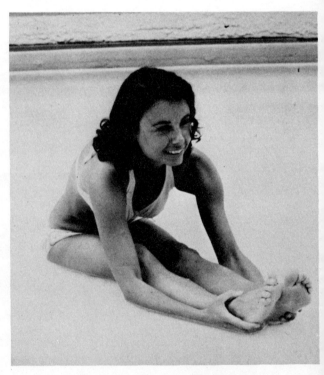

Figure 10-6

Head to Knee

Cat

—stretches your legs and spine
—reduces your abdomen

Sit with your legs together straight in front of you.

Inhale, stretching your arms overhead and leaning backward slightly.

Exhale, bending forward to clasp whatever part of your legs you can reach. Keep your head up. (Figure 10-6)

Repeat three times.

—prevents or corrects a rounded back
—relieves tension in your spine

Sit with your knees bent to your chest, your feet on the floor and one hand holding your other wrist in front of your knees. Hug your knees tightly to your chest.

Inhale, lifting your chest and straightening your spine as you drop your head back.

Exhale, rounding your back like a cat as you bring your forehead to your knees. Contract your abdomen.

Repeat three times.

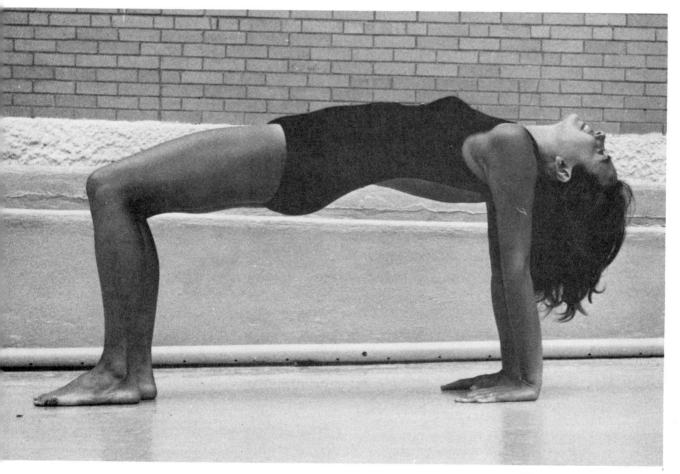

Figure 10-7

Bridge

Backward Bend

—strengthens your lower back and arms
Sit with your knees bent and your feet on the floor. Place your hands on the floor under your shoulders with fingers pointing forward.

—provides a therapeutic stretch to your feet, thighs, and spine
From a kneeling position, sit back on your heels. Place your hands on the floor behind your feet with your fingers pointing back.

Inhale, raising your hips from the floor until they are level with your knees. Let your head drop back. (Figure 10-7)

Inhale, raising your chest by arching your upper back. Remain seated on your heels.

Exhale, returning to a sitting position.

Exhale, dropping your head back. (Figure 10-8)

Repeat three times.

Repeat three times.

Figure 10-8

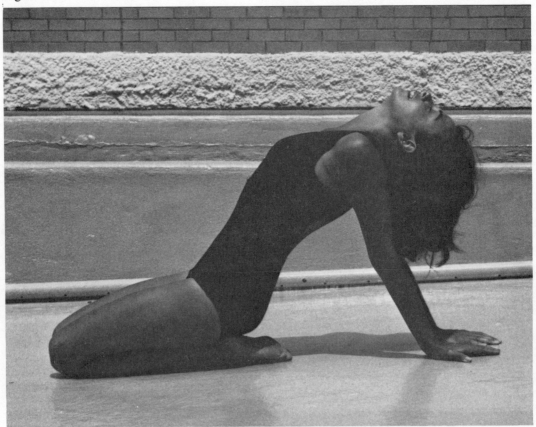

Backward Bend on Curled Toes

—provides a therapeutic stretch to your toes, thighs, and spine
From a kneeling position, curl your toes so they are pointing forward. Gradually put your weight on your heels until you can sit without difficulty on them for six seconds. Then proceed with the rest of the exercise by placing your hands behind you with your fingers pointing back.

Inhale, arching your back.

Exhale, dropping your head back. (Figure 10-9)

Figure 10-9

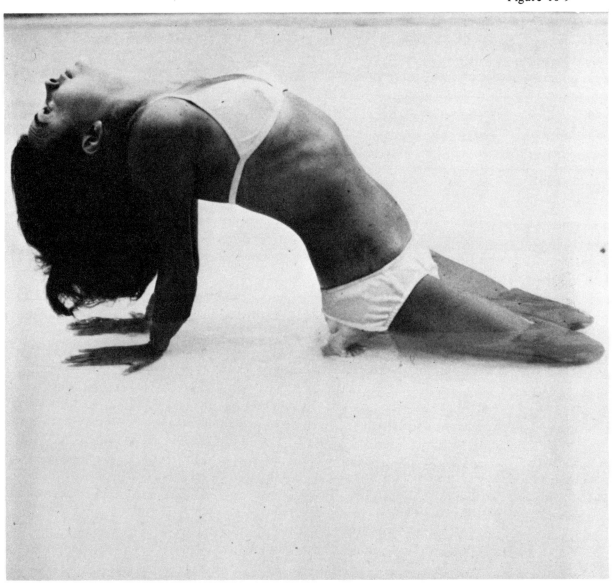

Slowly return to an upright position and repeat three times.
Advanced Variation: In the final position, gently walk your knees forward and back several inches for an extra stretch in your toes and feet.

Camel

   —improves your posture
   —increases your spinal flexibility

From a kneeling position, reach back and clasp your heels. Gently push your abdomen forward to arch your spine. Drop your head back, (Figure 10-10) Hold for as long as you are comfortable. Carefully return to a kneeling position by lifting your head up and using your back muscles to raise your body to a kneeling position again.

Repeat three times.

Figure 10-10

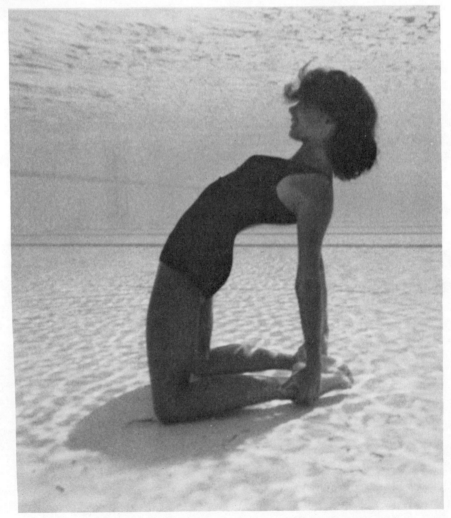

The Camel can also be done under water in the pool. From a standing position, reach back and clasp the front of both feet. Let your body submerge until you are kneeling on the pool floor. Keep your head up. (Figure 10-10)

Resistance Twist
—provides a therapeutic twist to your spine
—relieves tension in your shoulder blade area
Sit with your legs together straight in front of you. Twist your torso to the right
Inhale, pushing against the side with the tub or wading pool.

Inhale, pushing against the side with your right hand while pulling with your left hand. Look back over your right shoulder. Concentrate on the twisting stretch in your spine.

Exhale, relaxing your grip.

Repeat three times on each side.
This gentle twisting motion is a good warm - up for the more difficult exercise, the Twist.

Elbow to Knee

—trims your waistline
—relieves tension in your spine
Sit with your legs straight in front of you and your hands interlaced behind your head.

Inhale, pressing your head and elbows backward.

Exhale, twisting your trunk to the left and bending your left knee to meet your

right elbow. Look back under your left arm.

Continue by straightening your left leg, twisting to the right and bending your right knee to your left elbow.
Repeat six times to each side.

Modified Twist

—trims your waistline
—relieves tension in your spine
Sit with your legs straight in front of you. Cross your left foot over your right leg and place it on the floor outside your right knee. Hook your right arm over your left knee and grasp the outside of your right calf. Wrap your left arm behind your waist with your palm facing back.
Gently twist your torso and head back to the left. (Figure 10-11) Hold for a comfortable duration before slowly untwisting.
Repeat three times to each side.

Twist

—trims your waistline
—provides a therapeutic twisting stretch to your spine
This position may be too awkward for you to do in the bath. In that case, follow the same directions either in a wading pool or on land.
Sit with your back erect and both legs stretched out in front of you. Place your

Figure 10-11

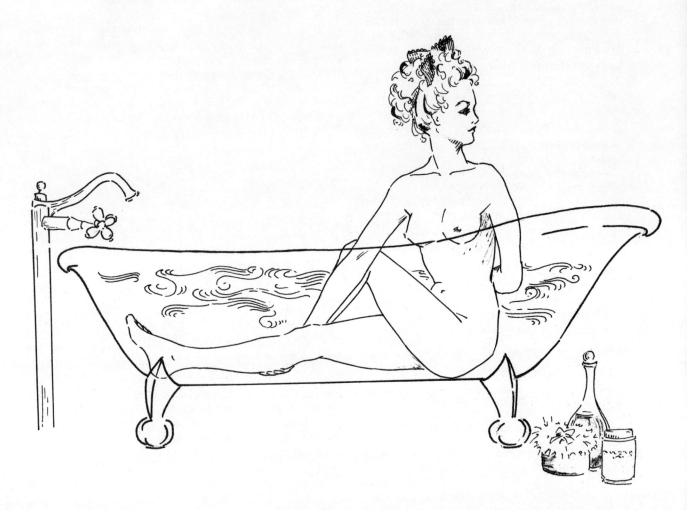

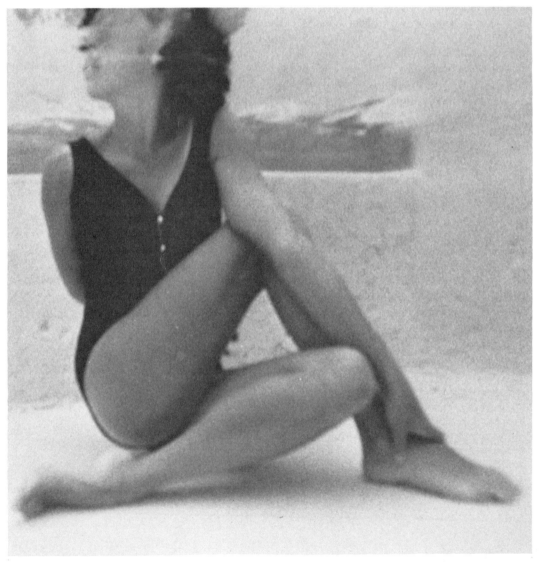

Figure 10-12

right foot on the floor beside the outside of your left knee. Bring your left foot to the right with the heel of your left foot under your right thigh. Hook your left arm over your right knee so that your left hand can grasp either your left knee or your right foot, whichever is more comfortable. Keep your spine erect even though you are leaning forward slightly.

Inhale, raising your right arm forward to shoulder level.

Exhale, twisting your head, torso and arm back to the right. Bend your right elbow and clasp the left side of your waist with your right hand. Keep your head up and look over your right shoulder to insure a gentle twisting and stretching of your entire spine. (Figure 10-12)

Hold this position for as long as you are comfortable; then slowly untwist to the starting position. Repeat on the other side by bringing your left foot over your right knee and your right foot to the left. Hook your right arm over your left knee and twist back with your left arm. Repeat three times on each side.
This ingenious posture, although sometimes difficult to do in the beginning, twists your spine in a unique, but natural, way, a way not generally a part of your daily activities. Your lower spine is locked into position so that your middle and upper spine can stretch and twist like a chain.

Lion

—helps prevent and eliminate facial wrinkles such as crow's feet
—provides temporary relief for sore throats
—tones, relaxes, and increases circulation in your face

From a kneeling position, sit on your heels with the palms of your hands resting on your knees.
Gently push your palms down on your knees and spread your fingers far apart. Simultaneously open your mouth and eyes as wide as possible and stretch your tongue out and down as if to touch your chin. Concentrate on tensing every muscle in your face and neck.
Hold for as long as you are comfortable (thirty seconds is the longest duration necessary), and then slowly bring your tongue back into your mouth, release all the tension in your face and neck, and rest your hands limply on your thighs. Enjoy the relaxed, refreshed feeling in your face.
Repeat three times.
You can do the Lion throughout the day when you feel tension building in your face, although it is especially effective in a steamy bath with a softening cream on your face.

Eye Exercises

—strengthen your eye muscles
—relieve tension and fatigue throughout your body

For all of the following exercises, relax in any comfortable position and imagine big clock in front of you. Move only your eyes to look at the imaginary numbers of the clock; your head remains still. Repeat each exercise three times, closing your eyes after each one to rest them.

1. Look far up to twelve o'clock and then straight down to six.
2. Look far over to nine and then across to three.
3. Circle your eyes by looking up at twelve, over to three, down to six and up to nine and twelve again. Reverse the rotation.

4. Look from twelve to nine to twelve to three; then from six to nine to six to three.

5. Look from one to seven to five to eleven and back to one again. Reverse by looking from one to eleven to five to seven and back to one again.

For a soothing, after - exercise treatment, apply alternate cold and warm washcloths to your closed eyes.

Chapter 11
Practice Schedules

The following programs are suggested combinations of exercises which offer a variety of movements possible within a fifteen to twenty minute period. As a beginner you may find a set routine helpful. As the exercises become more familiar to you, you can incorporate preferred ones into a more relaxed schedule, tailoring your own program to suit your individual needs. However you decide to do the exercises, be sure your sequence includes the following: (1) a few warm - ups (for endurance); (2) several forward, backward, sideward, and twisting stretches (for flexibility); and (3) several appropriate spot reducing exercises. The stretching movements are repeated two or three times. The warm - up and spot reducing exercises can be repeated more often with twenty the maximum number necessary. The repetitions and time spans suggested for each exercise are only approximate and need not be rigidly observed.

Those desiring only a mild form of exercise should begin with the Beginners' Program, keeping all movements slow and relaxed. Gradually add more inten- sive stretches from the Intermediate and Advanced levels. Avoid fatigue by relaxing between exercises and by ending your AQUAYOGA session when you are pleasantly tired. Your own limitations are your best guide to how much you should do.

To attain the peak of physical fitness and natural beauty possible, make a twenty to thirty minute exercise period as much a part of your daily routine as brushing your teeth. Many of the AQUAYOGA exercises can be done out of the water when no pool or lake is available. In addition to these, a program of basic yoga exercises is included for on - land practice. When using the following schedules, refer to the directions for each exercise for suggested timing and number of repetitions.

Let each AQUAYOGA session be an oasis of peace for you as you feel your body becoming more flexible, trim, relax- ed. Stretch your body in pure delight while taking long, deep, beautiful breaths. Lift yourself up to a look of grace and confidence. Listen to the small silences within you. Let the sun shine in!

Level I—Beginners (fifteen to twenty minutes)

		On-Land Variation	Page Number
Warm-Ups	Raised Leg Walk	X	25
	Knee Lift	X	26
	Flutter Kick		28
	Hopping		32
Stretches			
Forward	Wall Stretch		40
	Wall Walk		40
Backward	Half Locust	X	43
	Cobra	X	44
Twisting	Zig-Zag Walk	X	53
	Toe Twist	X	54
Sideward	Side Bend	X	60
	Hip Lift	X	60
Spot Reducers			
Arms, Shoulders, and	Shoulder Circling	X	65
Chest	Arm Rotation	X	66
	Pendulum Swing	X	66
Abdomen and Waistline	Arm Lifts	X	73
	Backward Arm and Leg Swing	X	73
	Knee Raises	X	74
Hips, Buttocks, and	Leg Crisscross	X	84
Thighs	Rapid Leg Lifts	X	85
Wrists, Hands, and	Thumb Stretch	X	94
Fingers	Thumb Circling	X	95
	Finger Stretch	X	95
	Hand Tenser	X	95
Knees	Knee Slap	X	96
Ankles, Feet, and Toes	Heel Flex	X	97
	Foot Side Stretch	X	97
Deep Relaxation		X	9

Level II—Beginners (fifteen to twenty minutes)

		On-Land Variation	Page Number
Warm-Ups	Jogging	X	26
	Leg Pushouts		29
	Side Jump		33
Stretches			
Forward	Wall Stretch		40
	Wall Walk		40
Backward	Cobra	X	44
	Elbow and Leg Lift	X	47
Twisting	Elbow to Knee	X	54
	Horizontal Twist	X	54
Sideward	Hip Lift	X	60
	Overhead Stretch	X	60
Spot Reducers			
Arms, Shoulders, and Chest	Horizontal Arm Swing	X	66
	Arc Swing	X	67
Abdomen and Waistline	Alternate Leg Raises	X	74
	Leg Crossover	X	74
	Leg Stretch	X	76
Hips, Buttocks, and Thighs	Side Arm and Leg Swing	X	85
	Alternate Leg Circling	X	85
	Leg Figure Eights	X	85
Wrists, Hands, and Fingers	Thumb Stretch	X	94
	Thumb Circling	X	95
	Finger Stretch	X	95
	Hand Tenser	X	95
Knees	Knee Slap	X	96
	Charleston	X	96
Ankles, Feet, and Toes	Heel Flex	X	97
	Foot Side Stretch	X	97
Deep Relaxation		X	**9**

Level III—Intermediate (fifteen to twenty minutes)

		On-land Variation	Page Number
Warm-Ups	Soldier Walk	X	27
	Foot Variations	X	28
	Bicycle Kick	X	29
	Leaping	X	33
Stretches			
Forward	Head to Knee	X	41
Backward	Locust	X	47
	Opposite Arm and Leg Bow	X	47
Twisting	Crocodile Series	X	55,101
Sideward	Hip to Wall	X	62
	Elbow Side Stretch	X	62
Spot Reducers			
Arms, Shoulders, and Chest	Arm Crossover	X	67
	Arm Circling	X	67
	Elbow Rotation	X	69
Abdomen and Waistline	Leg Lifts	X	76
	Wall Crawl		76
	Head to Knee Swing		76
Hips, Buttocks, and Thighs	Forward Arm and Leg Swing	X	87
	V Stretch	X	87
	Foot Figure Eights	X	87
Wrists, Hands, and Fingers	Wrist Bend	X	95
	Wrist Side Stretch	X	95
	Wrist Rotation	X	95
Knees	Knee Slap	X	96
	Knee Bend	X	96
Ankles, Feet, and Toes	Ankle Rotation	X	97
	Toe Bend	X	97
Deep Relaxation		X	9

Level IV—Intermediate (fifteen to twenty minutes)

		On-Land Variation	Page Number
Warm-Ups	Skipping	X	28
	Butterfly	X	31
	Split Jump		34
Stretches			
Forward	Head to Knee	X	41
Backward	Back Stretch		48
	Cat	X	49
Twisting	Crocodile Series	X	55, 101
	Standing Twist	X	54
Sideward	Hip to Wall	X	62
	Elbow Side Stretch	X	62
Spot Reducers			
Arms, Shoulders, and	Backward Elbow Jump	X	69
Chest	Elbow Jump	X	69
	Arm Glide	X	69
	Arm Figure Eights	X	69
Abdomen and Waistline	Wall Crossovers		77
	Body Stretch		77
	Alternate Toe Touch	X	78
Hips, Buttocks, and	Leg Circling	X	87
Thighs	Side Leg Raise	X	89
	Hip Rotator	X	89
Wrists, Hands, and	Wrist Bend	X	95
Fingers	Wrist Side Stretch	X	95
	Wrist Rotation	X	95
Knees	Knee Slap	X	96
	Knee Bend	X	96
Ankles, feet, and Toes	Ankle Rotation	X	97
	Toe Bend	X	97
Deep Relaxation		X	9

Level V—Advanced (twenty to twenty-five minutes)

Level VI— Advanced (twenty to twenty-five minutes)

		On-Land Variation	Page Number
Warm-Ups	Backward Kick	X	31
	Scissors Kick	X	32
	Forward Lunge		37
	Sideward Lunge		38
Stretches			
Forward	Ankle to Forehead	X	41
	Eagle	X	42
Backward	Bow	X	51
	Arm and Leg Stretch	X	52
	Swan	X	52
Twisting	Chest Expansion Twist	X	58
	Half Lotus Twist	X	60
Sideward	Triangle	X	63
	Lunge and Stretch	X	63
Spot Reducers			
Arms, Shoulders, and	Backward Hand Clasp	X	72
Chest	Prayer Position	X	73
Abdomen and Waistline	Tree	X	83
	Abdominal Lift	X	84
	Hip Swing		84
Hips, Buttocks, and	Pendulum Leg Swing		93
Thighs	Bent Knee Lift	X	94
	Bent Knee Balance	X	94
Wrists, Hands, and	Finger Fan	X	95
Fingers	Finger Flick	X	95
	Wrist Flick	X	96
Knees	Knee Slap	X	96
	Can-Can	X	97
Ankles, Feet, and Toes	Curled Toes Stretch	X	98
	Toe Fan	X	98
Deep Relaxation		X	9

For Swimmers Only (ten to fifteen minutes)

		On-Land Variation	Page Number
Stretches			
Forward	Child's Pose	X	100
	Head to Knee	X	106
Backward	Arm and Leg Lift	X	100
	Boat	X	101
	Backward Somersault		107
	Bow	X	108
Twisting	Crocodile Series	X	55,101
Sideward	Side Stretch	X	102
Spot Reducers			
Arms, Shoulders, and Chest	Hands to Shoulders		102
Abdomen and Waistline	V Arm and Leg Stretch		102
Hips, Buttocks, and	Scissors Kick	X	102
Thighs	Scissors Turn		104
	Head Stand Split	X	109
	Knee Bend		105
Deep Relaxation		X	9

Exercises for the Bath or Wading Pool (fifteen to twenty minutes)
They all can be done on land as directed

On-Land Hatha Yoga Program (fifteen to twenty minutes)

INDEX